NOVEMBER DAYS
A Love Story

by Bonnie Ruth

Frances Scott Press
Denver, Colorado

Copyright © 1995 by Bonnie Mary Ruth
All rights reserved
including the right of reproduction
in whole or in part in any form

Published by
Frances Scott Press
3801 E. Florida Ave., Suite 705
Denver, CO   80210

Cover design by
Debbie Rainguet

Printed in the United States of America

Publisher's Cataloging in Publication
(Prepared by Quality Books Inc.)

Ruth, Bonnie, 1942-
November days: a love story/by Bonnie Ruth. p.cm.
Preassigned LCCN: 95-92182.
ISBN 0-9645378-7-7

1. Young, Harl Henry, 1928-1989. 2. Ruth, Bonnie,
1942- 3. Cerebrovascular disease--Patients--Biography.
I. Title.

RC388.5.R88 1995   616.8'1'0092
                                   QBI95-20223

To Harl

This story is as true as I could tell it. Only some names have been changed.

Not yesterday I learned to know

The love of bare November days

Before the coming of the snow,

But it were vain to tell her so,

And they are better for her praise.

--Robert Frost

CHAPTER ONE

What region of the earth is not full of our calamities?
---Virgil

    Harl had begun to be ill about five days before. He thought he had the flu. Over the weekend his temperature started climbing, topping 102°. His right hand, long an annoyance to him because of poor circulation, was much worse; he constantly rubbed or shook it, scowling with the irritation of a man betrayed by the aging of his own body. He did not have a sore throat, but his voice had lost its power and came through as a whisper.
    He was fifty-four, with a distinguished career behind him, now a psychologist and professor and looking forward to gradual retirement. It would be a tranquil future in which he would write, maybe see a few patients, perhaps still teach a class here and there. But mostly slow down and enjoy himself; as he liked to say, "Watch the grass grow."
    We had lived together for five years, since shortly after the insertion of his plastic heart valve.
    I stood in front of or sat beside him, mountain casual in jeans and T-shirt, at forty-one an embodiment of the careless good health Harl with his lifelong heart problem wanted so badly to have. I said, *Call a doctor.*
    He was stubborn; he did not want to bother his doctor on a weekend. He whispered that he would cancel his appoint-

ments and see Dr. Friedman on Monday.

Harl in his bathrobe, I with veiled eyes bringing him water he sips, food he cannot eat. I said *Call a doctor call a doctor*, but I did not say how really frustrated I was. Nor did I simply pick up the phone and call the doctor myself. It was not for me to do that within the relationship Harl and I had, with much more difficulty than we ever expected, forged for ourselves in these five years of living together. He did not understand my feeling about an imbalance of power between us, my complaint that I felt no power to change him on anything. But didn't this whole weekend demonstrate exactly that?

Look back and wonder: How could I be more frightened of offending him than of what this illness might be doing to him?

* * *

Dr. Friedman told him to go into the hospital right away, for what seemed to be either pneumonia or possibly an infection at the site of the artificial heart valve. Harl by then was so ill that he had spent Monday morning sleeping in his desk chair, but he drew back as if Dr. Friedman had personally insulted him. He said, "I can't do that, Murray. I have a meeting tonight, and I have things to do at the school."

They bargained like two bankers closing a deal; Harl finally said he would go into the hospital Tuesday afternoon.

We stopped for dinner at a Japanese restaurant. I watched him from across the table, a man clearly very ill, wan and haggard and profoundly frightened. But if he was so frightened, why would he not go to the hospital? And as a psychologist with a specialty in couples and family treatment, why could he not see how frustrated I would be by his dismissal of my wishes at times like this?

In the difficult early years of our living together, he had started calling me "non-nurturing." The word had become a sore spot between us, the more so because, not understanding it, I was terrified by it. Were my feelings of that weekend evidence that I was non-nurturing? Did my anger now mean I was non-nurturing?

Harl realized only as I drove him home, with a frustrated giving-up movement of his hand, that he could not go to the meeting. It was his last as a member of the Board of Directors of the Jefferson County Mental Health Association; he had resigned as part of his ongoing resolution to work less. Tonight he was to be presented a plaque in honor of his service.

He called from the phone in our bedroom, whispering into the mouthpiece. "Hey, I've got this bug. I hate it, but I can't come tonight."

I could hear him laugh softly as someone answered; he said, "Thanks. Thanks, I will."

* * *

We were reading in bed. He laid down his book and put a hand on me, the hand cold, his face drawn. He said, "Bonnie, I don't think I have been doing very well these last months."

The heart surgery had been very hard on him, leaving him weak for at least a year. But that was five years ago, and it was in these last months that he had joined me in my rehabilitation counseling company, becoming our psychological consultant. Perhaps it was because that shared project made us feel closer, and both therefore happier, that I had perceived him as also feeling physically stronger.

I said, "I've thought you were getting better. What do you mean?"

He looked off across the room to consider that, his face showing instantly the thoughtful considering look that was so habitual to it. I waited for him to answer, and after a while closed my eyes. I did not realize I dozed, or know that the Harl I knew had spoken his last words to me.

* * *

It was the oddness of a sound that brought me awake: Harl's head tapping against our bedroom door. He was lying on the floor, seeming semi-conscious but not speaking. I thought he had fainted; I pulled him up in my arms and tried to wake him.

His body rolled against me, his head falling forward like a rag doll's. He made no sound but tightened his left arm around me, as if in that frantic terrified grip he had found his only communication.

In the ambulance I turned my seat around to watch the heart monitor, expecting it to go dark at any moment. Harl was awake but would not speak or even shake his head for "yes" or "no." An attendant told him to blink his eyes once for "yes" and twice for "no." Then he asked him if he was in pain anywhere, and Harl carefully blinked his eyes twice. No.

We had all thought it was a heart attack. The word *stroke* was now forming in my mind.

At the hospital nurses and residents instantly surrounded him, taping electrodes all over him, rushing him into Intensive Care. Someone asked me if I was his wife. A sign on the door said only family members could come in. I said yes, feeling suddenly the shock of my non-status. They could keep me out; I did not technically have a right to be here.

Everyone but I knew what to do. The nurses had him into a hospital gown and hooked to a heart monitor in minutes. Residents hung over him, listening to his heart and asking him questions. He stared at everyone and made no answer.

Some of the crowd cleared out while waiting for Dr. Friedman. I went to Harl then and reached across his chest to hug him, my cheek nestling next to his. There was the familiar hollow between his cheek and throat, his warm familiar scent. His left arm tightened again around me, and I felt the terror in his grip.

Dr. Friedman found me in the waiting room to tell me it seemed to be a stroke. No one else had told me anything.

He asked, "Are you and Harl married now?"

They had told him I said we were. He knew we had not been before. I flooded with relief at no longer having to lie, while also registering the absurdity of taboos like this at such a time.

"No, I just told them that. I was afraid they wouldn't let me in."

Dr. Friedman must have fixed it with whoever was in charge, because after that no one called me Mrs. Young anymore, but they did let me in.

A nurse came when Dr. Friedman had gone and asked me kindly if I would like to sleep in a vacant patient room. That surprised me because I had thought it was "not done." In times of shock, notions of propriety can take over and get us through. I would not have questioned being left all night in the waiting room.

Alone on the hospital bed, I tried to grasp that this was real, that nothing was ever going to be the same again. I had always envied Harl his ability to cry easily, at a moving play, a patient making a breakthrough, a child hitting a home run. My own tears came hard, forced into the flat hospital pillow by my knowing I must admit that much reality, must do that much for myself.

* * *

I woke at three in the morning, anxiety engulfing me. The nurse had said I could sleep here, but what if by now the shift had changed and no one knew where I was? I could not wait for the elevator; I ran down the stairs and pushed open the door to Intensive Care.

He was sleeping now, hooked to the monitors and myriad I.V. tubes, his ragged breathing saying he was still alive. Harl.

His face was oddly rigid in sleep. In other times that had been a face of extraordinary expressiveness, blue eyes lit with love or shrewd with swift perception.

Harl sitting up in bed mornings to watch me dress, smiles flitting across his face at each stage of the transformation, never tiring of the miracles of makeup and curling iron and clothes he had encouraged me to buy, until the moment when I would turn to him a polished capable businesswoman and he would laugh for the sheer joy of it.

Harl coming home evenings tired from his long days of work, never with foul temper or discouragement but instead with optimism for our evening, starting dinner if it was his turn to cook, sitting with drinks on the deck to enjoy the mountain air and ask, eyes lighting with that special look they had for me and speaking with humorous mild irony at the banality of the question, "And how was *your* day?"

Harl with a suitcase and plane tickets in his hand, radiant because we are leaving for the airport and he will get to show me Hawaii, where he has been but I have not.

Harl sitting beside me in bed on a Sunday morning, laying down his newspaper to take my hand and say as he has said before, always with the same mix of puzzlement and pleasure, "I don't think you *know* how lovely you are."

Back in the too-bright hospital corridors, I began to roam. I knew I would not sleep again this night. It had been two years since I smoked, but suddenly I was craving a cigarette.

I went outside and walked a block to an all night Safeway. This was a rough neighborhood, close to downtown. The glare of heedless auto lights seemed suited to my own internal landscape, desolated by the careless violence of an uncaring universe.

I would have to call Harl's family, and the professional school where he taught, and the psychology group with whom he practiced. I had already called my children, who had gotten up in the night to run and stand at the end of our driveway so the ambulance would not miss our mountain home, but I would have to call them again. I would have to call someone to take me home, because I had come down in the ambulance with Harl and had no transportation.

I would have to call my office, the office Harl shared with me, and tell them--

Tell them what?

I could call no one now, at this hour. I dropped my quarters in the cigarette machine and began to let my mind move cautiously forward, to encompass just this night and nothing else: I would sit in the hospital coffee shop drinking coffee and smoking cigarettes until morning, and then I would go into one of the pay phone booths and begin calling everyone.

Beyond that I had no idea what my life or Harl's would be like, from now on.

* * *

Harl was still sleeping at five but awake at seven, his weak smile saying he knew me. I reached through the side bars of his bed to hold his hand.

He did not make a sound.

A doctor came in, crisp in his white jacket. He said, "I'm Dr. Iminoff, the neurologist," and did a quick examination, shining a light into Harl's eyes, tapping him for reflexes. Then he leaned over to look him clearly in the eyes and said in a loud voice, "Harl, we think you've had a stroke."

Harl grimaced and nodded. His eyes looked entirely comprehending.

Dr. Iminoff's eyes flicked over me. He asked, "Are you his wife?"

I answered truthfully this time. "No, I live with him."

Dr. Iminoff lowered his eyes and never really talked to me again.

Harl's treatment was what mattered; I could put up with one cold fish doctor. As with almost everything else I ever had to cope with, I had something Harl had once said to me to help me. He had been talking about his second wife's treatment for multiple sclerosis, and said that neurologists were a different breed from other doctors: "Most doctors are in it for the love"--he had a way of gesturing as he talked, this time as if rifling money, with a movement of it in toward his heart--"the love they get for curing people. But neurologists spend most of their time telling people they have terrible incurable diseases."

His expression had indicated some distaste but also the acceptance that made him so gifted as a psychologist. He said, "It takes a different kind of person."

Dr. Friedman had been Harl's cardiologist for twenty years and would talk to me. I stood with him a few hours later outside the patient room where he was having Harl transferred, my horror beginning to take the form of *why*.

Harl was only fifty-four; why would he have had a stroke?

Dr. Friedman spoke from behind his pince-nez glasses in his usual soft and very professional, yet kindly way. "What we think is that he may have had the flu, and the bug got into his bloodstream and caused an infection at the site of his artificial heart valve. Then blood clots from there were thrown into the bloodstream and went to his brain, and caused the stroke."

What was coming was worse.

"The valve is almost certainly going to have to be replaced. It's like an abscess; you can't treat it with antibiotics only, and we are afraid that if the infection is allowed to continue, he could have another stroke. But right now he is so weakened by the stroke that we are afraid he could not survive the surgery.

"So we want to postpone it as long as we can, and give him time to regain some strength. We will stand by and keep listening to the valve, and if it seems to be slipping, we will have to do the surgery."

Dr. Friedman also advised me to try to continue life as usual, but such a thing was not possible. If this had been the heart problem only, maybe--but this was Harl unable to talk or perhaps even think; wouldn't he need me to be with him?

Through that day and the next he slept or sat propped on pillows in his blue hospital gown. The stroke had not affected his face too badly; the right side drooped only a little, and his smile was just a little crooked. He did smile. He smiled at the nurses who brought him food, and broadly at me each time I came in. He fed himself, though very oddly. He would eat with a knife, or dip mashed potatoes in his grape juice.

I ran back to the Safeway to buy him a pen and notebook. His right hand was completely paralyzed, but he was left-handed and so hopefully could write.

He took the pen eagerly and wrote:

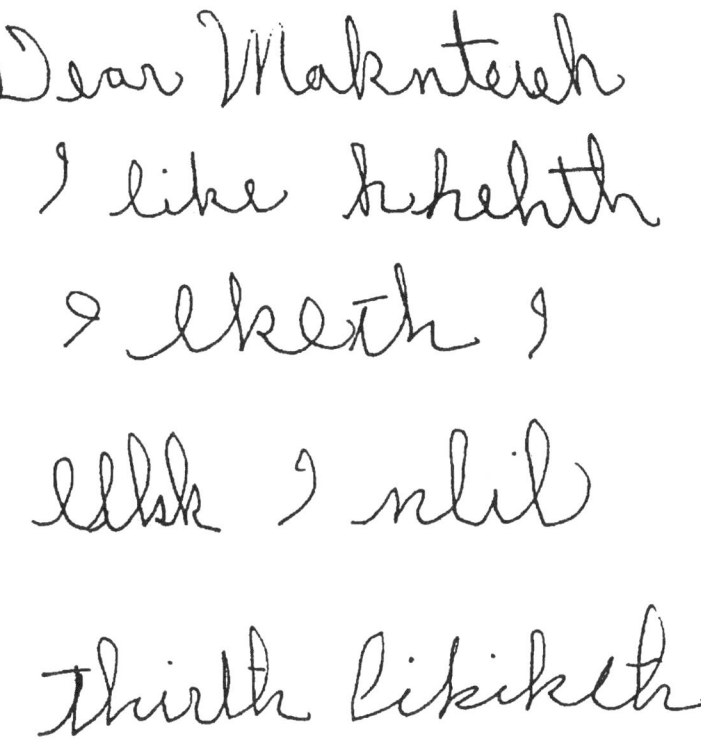

What could it be like for him from the inside, his mind shattered, the words with which he wanted to think not there to think with? As a psychologist he knew a lot about the brain; he must know he had had a stroke. What was he feeling?

The hospital had regular prescribed visiting hours, but when Dr. Friedman saw I needed to stay, he let me. I sat on a chair in a corner, where I could stare at Harl as the hours went by and his fever went up. He was very sick.

And he still did not make a sound.

* * *

New words fell like puzzle pieces around us: *apraxia, perseveration.*

A doctor said, "Harl, open your mouth."

Harl stared hard at him, the same baffled stare he had given the ambulance attendants when they asked him questions. He did not open his mouth.

I said eagerly helpful, "I *know* he can open his mouth. He does it to eat."

But the doctor was shaking his head. "That's different; that is a motor function. What he can't do is follow a command, voluntarily initiate the action. It's called *apraxia.*"

Now he said, "Harl, touch your ear," and Harl at once touched his ear.

This was too mystifying. I said as if the doctor were responsible, "Why can he touch his ear if he can't open his mouth?"

"Because he has *oral apraxia.* Basically it means he can't voluntarily open his mouth."

To Harl he said, "Harl, touch your ear again," and Harl who had kept his hand on his ear slowly took it off and put it back again.

The doctor said, "Again," and he did it again.

But when the doctor said, "Now touch your shoulder," he continued to touch his ear.

The doctor nodded, as if this were what he had expected. He said, "That is *perseveration.* It means his mind gets stuck; he can't switch it."

As in his attempts to write notes, the hopeless repetitions of letters.

Everyone had been telling me Harl's voice would come

back, when some of the swelling of his brain went down. But no one knew how damaged his speech would be. This doctor said, "The worst, and I'm afraid the longest lasting form of apraxia, is usually verbal apraxia, the inability to initiate words."

He gently moved Harl's hand from his ear to his shoulder and said again, "Harl, touch your *shoulder*."

And Harl who had kept looking at him practically without blinking began touching his shoulder.

A nurse came in with an electric razor and propped a mirror on his bed table. It was the third morning since the stroke, and she was going to let him shave himself. She said when I murmured astonishment, "Shaving is a motor task. Motor tasks aren't usually affected by a stroke."

He could not open his mouth on command, but he could pick up a razor and shave.

More importantly he saw his reflection, and suddenly lit up. He was happy anyway because I had come for breakfast and because he liked being allowed to shave, but now he smiled delight at me, gesturing, turning his head to examine his face.

What must it be like for him from the inside, with the thoughts by which he knew himself gone, that it would make him this happy to see the simple intactness of his face?

He was still shaving when a team of students arrived. These teams came in several times a day, encircling his bed, all carrying clipboards on which they wrote furious notes. I listened always from my seat in the corner, watching Harl between their white-coated backs. Today he watched them so intently it seemed his face must crack.

Did they know how intelligent he was, how much knowledge lay behind that intent listening face?

A young woman listened through a stethoscope to his

heart murmur and exclaimed, "I never heard one that loud before!"

Unlike Dr. Friedman and the nurses, who were always careful what they said in front of Harl, these student teams seemed to think that because he could not talk, he could not hear. But did they also think I could not hear?

The resident in charge agreed that the murmur was one of the worst he had ever heard and began explaining about the impending surgery.

Dr. Friedman had not been telling Harl about the surgery, thinking it might upset him too much. I did not know whether Harl had already grasped what they were saying or not, but I interrupted, as politely as I could.

"Excuse me, but his doctor said not to tell him about the surgery."

They stopped but looked at me as if I were crazy. It had not occurred to them he could hear, or that it mattered if he did. The resident lowered his eyes in the manner of Dr. Iminoff. I was not supposed to be here at this hour anyway, and I had embarrassed him in front of his students. They filed out without saying a word to me.

At once I was blaming myself: not that I had spoken but that I did not handle confrontations well, that Harl if our roles had been reversed, I lying helpless on the bed and he there to protect me, would have managed it ever so much better. I could imagine exactly how, although I could not mimic him. Rather than the single sentence left hanging like a bomb in the air, Harl would have given them some interaction. He would have moved into the group and said comfortably, "Hey, she might hear you. Let's remember that, okay?" And no one would have been angry at him.

Before I could decide whether Harl had understood the comments about the surgery, Dr. Iminoff arrived, student in tow. The same student was always with him, a curly-haired young man on crutches who at least said hello to me, which Dr. Iminoff did not.

Dr. Iminoff lifted the blankets to examine Harl's paralyzed right side. He said to the student, with distaste, "This is *massive*."

There was an advantage to being seemingly invisible; Dr. Iminoff knew more than he had told me. This was the first time I had heard the word "massive" applied to Harl's stroke.

Dr. Iminoff had brushed off all my questions about recovery, saying he needed a CAT scan before he could make any predictions. I came out of my invisibility to ask about the CAT scan. Did he know yet when it would be done?

He snapped an instrument into his bag and answered as though I were being a nuisance. "No. If he survives the heart condition, then we'll worry about the stroke."

The student gave me a slightly worried look as they left.

Shocked to the bone, I looked at Harl to see if he had registered this. He had been watching Dr. Iminoff intently throughout, but gave no sign.

I resumed staring at him. Staring, and trying to imagine that one day soon the sun could rise on a world without him in it.

* * *

His parents and two sisters had come, the parents almost eighty and so frail that I did not see how they could survive this, or how Donna and Jeane could manage them.

We clustered in a waiting room trying to decide how best to work the visit. I had told Harl they were coming, but it still seemed that everyone probably should not drop in on him all at once.

Harl had grown up in small town Tennessee, the oldest child and only son of this family, his father a barber. He had told me how throughout their childhood he and Donna were constant companions, skinny dipping with other children in a creek, walking together in a parade each year: as he described it, "Hand in hand."

He also told me how as a self-important teenager he finally drove Donna away: "Well you see, I had my *things* to do."

And added with the look of a man who never underestimated the depth of such experiences, "I'm not sure if she ever forgave me."

Donna was fifty now, still small and blond and softly southern. She said perhaps she should not be the first one to walk in, so Jeane took their mother first. Harl smiled and nodded, stretching out his left hand since he could not move his right.

His father went in, and then Donna.

Harl made his first sound. He had started to smile at Donna, but all at once his face crumpled and a sound, a moan, began to force its way out of him. Once started it continued, anguished, the most terrible sound that could ever exist in the world. His face contorted with the physical pain of getting it out; his head tossed on the pillow. An animal making such a sound would be shot for kindness.

That was what it was like for him.

Nurses rushed in trying to help. He began to have a chill; doctors were paged and quickly converged around the bed; someone was bringing oxygen.

CHAPTER TWO

The beloved of my heart, my shelter and defense
Against the bleak south wind.
My speaking-bird that charmed the assembled tribes,
That swayed the people's councils.

---*Old Maori Lament*

His family had left, the parents too weak to stay long. Alone again, I roamed the hospital halls, or sat and stared at Harl, or smoked in the cafeteria. Almost two weeks had passed, and he had not yet had to have the surgery. But he still could not speak at all.

Telephones were my link to the world, the old lost world from before Harl's stroke. I dropped my quarter in and waited. Cathryn answered on the second ring, her voice lighting in fourteen-year-old delight: "Mom!"

But she was going to Christy's to spend the night. And David and Steve were just leaving for the evening too, so suddenly there was no reason for me to go home. The thought appalled me, the big empty house, all the reminders of Harl and nothing to do but think.

I could not be alone now, without at least the superficial proximity to people that I had here at the hospital. Days everyone thought I held up magnificently; I was so stoic that I surprised even myself. But evenings as I drove through dusk toward home I began to tremble, and nights I was sleeping with Harl's robe curled in my arms, for the scent of him.

I had stared at him so many hours that I still saw him when I closed my eyes to sleep: his face feverish, confused, but still welcoming me every time I came in; his eyes turning habitually to me as the hours passed, our communication more intense than speech.

I hung up the phone and went to the cafeteria, not for machine vended sandwiches this time but a real dinner, overcooked pot roast and boiled potatoes. Mostly hospital staff people ate in here; patient relatives hung out next door in the coffee shop where they could smoke and get the cheap sandwiches.

I left my dinner half eaten and went there, to have a cigarette with my coffee. The vacant-eyed people in the coffee shop were better to be around than the too-cheerful cafeteria crowd. I watched them covertly, the same people I kept passing in the elevators and hallways, all of us zombie-like from whatever had ripped our lives to land us here.

What was it Harl had said? When we were dating, when I used to drive to the moss-rocked duplex he had built for his crippled second wife, Dian. Beautiful Dian, whom I felt I knew.

Dian had been the worst mistake of Harl's life, their marriage a disaster even before she came down with the multiple sclerosis. She was utterly unstable, endlessly in therapy and always firing her therapists. Harl had smiled as he pantomimed her coming home from one of those sessions, a first and last with a woman psychologist: "You know what that bitch said to me? She said, 'Go home and love your husband!' Why, I'll have an affair anytime I want--that bitch--she said, 'Go home and love your husband!'"

His smile faded. He said, "She was a baby, I had a baby on my hands. And then when she got sick, I had a sick and crippled baby on my hands."

But with the multiple sclerosis he would not leave her. He cared for her for nine years at home before finally having to institutionalize her, and bore all the cost of the institutionalization.

What Harl had told me about caring for Dian was all I knew of my own position now, he suddenly an invalid, I the one to stand by him or not. I smoked, tapping ashes into the overflowing tinfoil ashtray, remembering.

He had described those nine years always with the same horror, Dian in a wheelchair with her beauty gone, desperately unhappy, endlessly demanding. "In a year we would go through a hundred housekeepers. A lot of them lasted only until lunchtime. I was down at the Division then"--what he called being down at the Division was being director of the Colorado Division of Mental Health--"and just about noon I'd get these calls from these women saying, 'I can't stand this, I'm leaving....'"

He was a marvelous talker, the way he put words together, the way he could mimic the speech of other people to convey so strong a sense of them that I felt I absolutely knew them. One of his students who came to visit him here at the hospital told me he had made History of Psychology sound like a fairy tale: "It was the highlight of the program, because Harl would act out all the parts."

But what exactly was it he had said about himself and Dian, about not being cynical?

I was hoarding his words now, wanting to remember them exactly right. I put out my second cigarette and went back to the elevator and up to his room, where he sat in the dim light looking at the television. He smiled as always when I came in; I sat down and reached through the bars to hold his hand. It felt hot, startling because his hands were usually cold from poor circulation. His fever must be going up.

Harl had said by the time he and I were living together that he had no love left for Dian. About that he was adamant: "None." But there was a tenderness in the way he talked about her, the way he often called her *poor child*.

"Poor child, she thought she wanted to kill herself, but she could never bring herself to do it. And then when physically she couldn't anymore, she started begging *me* to. And I might have, I thought about it. Except for the possibility of criminal charges. I really might have."

She had made her attempts. "Poor child, she thought she was trying, but she always bungled it. I would wake up and find her on the floor in the kitchen or bathroom with just the tiniest scratches on her wrists, and she would say in this pitiful little voice, 'I'm sorry, I couldn't do it.'"

His face darkened. He said, "Apologizing to *me* for *her* life."

I had been the one to take the call from the nursing home on the morning Dian died, guessing what it was even as I handed Harl the phone: complicity somehow even in the handling of the phone, a guilt spilling over from him. When he hung up, he began rushing between the bureau and the dresser, searching for handkerchiefs or car keys as if that was what mattered.

This was too much. I was supposed to be the one prone to denial. But here was Harl who had just been told his wife was dead, behaving as though this frenetic search for car keys was what was important. I went to him, put my arms around him and said, "Wait."

He breathed deeply then and said he did not know how to feel.

By then he had been paying twelve thousand dollars a year for six years to keep Dian comatose in the home; he and

I were living together and he thought he was ready for her to die. But that afternoon he found two dollar bills tucked away among her things, and he sat down and cried like a baby. It was the amount of money the home allowed its residents to have, and so she did.

We stared together at his hospital room television, a game show, lots of color and action. Was he understanding it? He seemed to get riveted to it, as if he could not pull his attention off it.

Harl riveted to a game show?

I was staring without seeing, still remembering. What exactly was it he had said? Something about Dian, something important to me now. I knew the general drift, but I wanted the exact words.

Harl's ambition as director of mental health had been to create a community-based mental health system, one of the nation's first. He succeeded, making that stunning success of his professional life even as his personal one lay in shambles. He was making mental health history, emptying out the State Hospital, shaping a system that many other states would make their model.

By the time we were dating he spoke of it with some ruefulness, recalling his own single-minded exercise of power. "I was going to do it, make that mental health system more humane. And I did, and there are a lot of people who don't like me. And I don't blame them."

But a lot of people did like him too, huge numbers of them: students, colleagues, patients and former patients streaming through the hospital. Flowers covered every available surface of this room; I had papered a wall with his get-well cards.

The messages people had written on some of those cards were poignant to me, testaments to Harl's special influence on their lives. I knew that mentoring quality in him; there was no one he had influenced more than me.

I was thirty-one when I met him, just six months out of the marriage I had entered at nineteen. My own history when we talked then sounded bleak in the telling, a mother who died, a preoccupied and distant father, a stepmother bad enough to send me into the equally bad early marriage. I had never flown in an airplane, or travelled anywhere except to my husband's parents' home in Oklahoma. *Unsophisticated* hardly describes it.

Worse than the superficial summary: my four sisters and I beggars, less than beggars because not allowed to speak, in a family of middle class affluence. I had not been provided a pair of school shoes between my father's marriage when I was fourteen and my own five years later; my sister Leslie still bears ugly lumps on her heels from a pair of ill-fitting shoes she bought with babysitting money at thirteen, and which were never replaced. Our stepmother hid the bandages and postage stamps so we would not be able to use them. We were not allowed to bring friends to our home. None of us was ever allowed to drive. We were not allowed in our own living room in the evenings; we would not have dreamed of turning on a radio or television.

Reality in the stepmother myth, but the myth not so much *Cinderella* as *Hansel and Gretel*: because of the sweet adored father who lets it happen. I would never in my life have a relationship not so complicated by warring feelings as nearly to rip it apart.

Harl forty-four and Director of Mental Health; I thirty-one in my twenty dollar polyester dresses, with warring feelings and three small children and looking for a job. What did he see in me, Harl who made the sun come up?

On our first date he had offered to take me to my favorite

restaurant, and I could not name one. I bluffed and said let's go to his favorite this time and mine next time, thinking that by next time I could find out the names of some restaurants.

We had dated briefly then, but not seriously until a couple of years later, when I was more ready. It was two years after that we moved to Evergreen together, and on our fifth anniversary of living together that I pulled him speechless from our bedroom floor.

An odor of diarrhea suddenly filled the hospital room. Intravenous antibiotics did this to him; he could not control it. Nurses repeatedly dropped whatever they were doing to come clean him up, never seeming to mind, always cheerful with him. Harl's awareness of what had happened fluctuated; sometimes he seemed hardly to realize.

This time he did. His face twisted as he tried in vain to lift his body out of it. His paralyzed right side would not let him move; he was so horrified that he managed to throw his left arm and leg over the right, almost pulling over his I.V. stand. I was afraid he would hurt himself; I put my hands on him and said to calm him, "Wait, I'll get the nurse."

Tonight's nurse was not one of Harl's regular nurses but a young man whom I had not met until he bounced in a few hours before, well-nourished and very full of himself, announcing that he was to be the relief nurse. Unlike the regular nurses, he did not talk at all about Harl but only about himself: how overworked he was, how much paperwork he had to do.

The resident on duty then and now was the one who disliked me for reminding him not to talk in front of Harl. This nurse had an air of camaraderie with him that the female nurses (I thought, the real nurses) did not. He had tooled in during rounds as the resident was listening to Harl's heart, to announce jovially of some other patient, "I can see why she was feeling faint. Her pulse is 150!"

A great joke. I stayed quiet, watching from the shadows of my corner, rage moving in me at the thought that they could talk about Harl that way. The resident smiled, finished with Harl and went out with him.

I found the nurse now in the hallway just outside Harl's room. He said he would come as soon as he finished with a patient in the next room.

Harl had started thrashing again. Again I calmed him with the promise of the nurse. "Lie still just a minute; he'll be *right* here."

Five minutes passed, ten. Harl waited with his forehead broken out in sweat, able to lie still only because I patted and soothed him. Finally I went back to look for the nurse again and found him seated at the station, drinking coffee and talking jovially with the resident.

I knew better; I knew I could only lose. Getting angry only lets them call you crazy. I should stay deferential, say something meek like, "Could you get to Harl soon?"

I said in seething outrage, "Come on!"

The nurse gestured in grandiose innocence to the heart monitors, speaking as one incredulously wounded. "I'm the only one on the monitors. I can't leave."

I knew very well that the real nurses would leave the monitors with the other person to go clean up a patient. Tonight the other person was the resident, sitting right there doing paperwork. Or was; now he had stopped to stare intently at me.

That the resident could watch the monitors for ten minutes was so obvious that I did not bother to argue about it. Instead I went viciously to the point: "So you're going to let him lie in his crap?"

It was the resident who answered. He said curtly, "That's

right."

Score one for the medical profession.

I had no power, nothing to threaten them with. Those two did not care if Harl lay in excrement all night. Where were the real nurses? I could think of nothing more impressive to do than say, "Then I'll clean him up myself," and whirl back to the room.

Which of course bothered them not at all. They were happy to let me clean him up myself; it meant they would not have to do it.

Harl was panting from the effort of waiting. I calmed myself enough to turn his eyes to me and tell him, wryly but gently, "Your *male nurse* is refusing to clean you up. I'm going to do it."

The look of sheer disbelief he gave me showed he had understood.

I managed it with towels from the bathroom, pulling a sheet from the other bed. By the time I was through Harl was exhausted, his head limp on the pillow, his cheeks hot. I turned off the television and laid my cheek against his, feeling the pulse in his temple. It was much too fast.

Only one other person was still in the coffee shop, a man in work clothes and a couple of days' stubble staring into his empty paper cup. My hands still trembled as I tried to light my cigarette. I should not have done it, lost control like that. What story would those two make of it?

Harl would have managed it better; he could wield power without losing control. I smoked, and tried again to remember just what it was that he had said. Something about Dian, and his patients, and disappointments.

Certainly he had had his share of disappointments. Barely five feet, five inches tall, he had nevertheless played first string football in high school and won an athletic scholarship.

Bursting with plans for himself, he next joined the Navy to get V.A. college benefits, then almost immediately came down with the rheumatic fever that damaged his heart valve, ended all athletics and confined him for a year to a military hospital.

He had told me with his usual gift for storytelling how that experience was what first got him interested in Psychology. "So I was in bed for a year, and I ran through everything in the military library, and there was a doctor who said I could use his private library. And I was making my way through everything in his library, and I came across this fellow named *Frude*."

Excited, he had tried to talk to the doctor about "this Frude fellow." He mimicked for me the doctor's frantic expression as he corrected him: "Hey, it's Freud, *Freud*...!"

Freud or Frude, Harl left that hospital eighteen years old and knowing he wanted to be a psychologist.

He also left with the damaged heart valve. Perhaps that was what made him love life so much, knowing his might be short.

The man was still staring into his cup when I went out. I walked past the elevators and all the way to others at the end of the corridor, then on each floor got off and walked back again. Working my way in that fashion back to Harl's room on the fifth floor, I dodged the nursing station and tiptoed in for a last time before starting home.

The scent of him was very strong, because of his fever. I watched him sleep and remembered at last the exact words he had said, as I sat by him listening and learning.

"I suppose I'm still narcissistic enough to have a lot of anger. When you're young and you're bright and you get a lot of attention for that, you can start thinking you're *special*. Then when life proceeds to knock you about the same as everyone else, you say"--he gestured in humorous outrage, arms extended toward the universe--'What's *this*?'"

His arms dropped back, his smile just a little rueful. "But what turns me off most in being a therapist is seeing how *greedy* people are. How they get married for all these things"--his gesture now was one of vague distaste--"all these things they think they're going to *get*. Then I hear all these men saying, 'Women are no good, you can't trust 'em, they'll take all your money'"--a gesture now indicating *on and on*--"and all these women saying, 'Men are no good, they'll use you and cheat on you....'

"And I think I've been through about the worst of that whole man/woman thing, I got all the bad parts and not much of the good, but I don't claim to dislike women and I am not bitter."

He said then the words I had remembered always, that I had been trying to get exactly right tonight.

"Patients nowadays mostly come in and say to me, 'Life stinks!' and I say, 'You're right!'"--here a laugh as he pantomimed his own emphatic agreement--"And I let them figure out, if they have it in them, that life is still all they have and they might as well give it the best they have."

He finished with a rich smile at me, his special look for me. He had been through the worst of it, but he was letting himself fall in love again, with me.

* * *

Monday morning and the CAT scan report was in. Dr. Iminoff was to be here at eleven-thirty to talk to me about it, following a conference with the other doctors. Harl was sleeping. Friends and I pulled chairs together in the hallway outside his room. Eleven-thirty came and went, then twelve. We talked and joked.

One of our group was a nurse from my office who knew something about hospital procedures. She said Dr. Iminoff had probably stayed for the lunch that followed the staff consult. She spoke to the nurses at the station, who called the consult room to tell him we were waiting.

Twelve-thirty, twelve forty-five, one o'clock. Our laughter had become strained. Just after one Dr. Iminoff arrived, tight-lipped and icy as always. I asked him what the CAT scan showed.

Dr. Iminoff threw me a look of the most extreme irritation. "You can't tell anything from a CAT scan. The therapy is what matters."

He strode on past us into the room.

We were stunned into silence. Dr. Iminoff had had me living for that report, and now he claimed it meant nothing. It must be very bad, and he did not care to talk to me about it.

My friends murmured about being sorry. They had to begin to leave.

I went back in to sit by Harl. He was grey-faced and not yet shaved, and seemed to want to go right back to sleep. I watched him doze, one side of his face stiff with paralysis. What everyone commented on about Harl, the
visitors who streamed in here and stopped to talk to me, was just what I had been recalling through my vigil of three nights before: his zest, his love of life, his spirit. The zest he could not have had if he had let himself be bitter, Harl sharing plates in a restaurant or smiling over an apron as he begins to cook; his love of people, good times, *fun*. Bubbles ran from the oxygen tank through the plastic tube to his nostrils; his lips that could not speak lay slightly parted. The CAT scan must be very bad; recovery would not be good. Oh Harl where has

all your fun gone now.

CHAPTER THREE

"What's happened to me?" he thought. It was no dream.

--Franz Kafka, <u>The Metamorphosis</u>

    A call from Dr. Friedman was waiting for me at my office. I had just left the hospital; he must have missed me by minutes. I pushed the phone buttons without sitting down, my eyes drifting unseeing over the piles of papers on my desk. A nurse answered; when I identified myself she said at once, "Oh," and paged Dr. Friedman.

    I knew then that the worst must have happened, though the breath still left me when Dr. Friedman said it. Harl's valve had slipped enough that they must do immediate surgery.

    I put the receiver down and stared vacantly at the wall for what seemed a long time but could only have been a few minutes. Then I went out to tell the other people here, the secretaries and counselors who worked for me. They knew Harl and cared for him; they were sorry this was happening to him and to me. But there was also in their eyes a question as to my ability to hold up, and what the consequences of that might be for them. They did not want me to fall apart; they did not want me to let this business go.

    Dr. Friedman and I stood in our usual spot in the hallway outside Harl's room while he explained to me. "The valve sounds definitely worse. We've all talked about it, and he's going to have to have the surgery. We'd rather wait till Monday when the operating room is better staffed, but he may need it sooner, and if he does we can handle that. We'll have to keep listening to the valve and be ready."

Harl must be told. I knew I was the one to do it. The city had darkened outside his window; I stood in the dim light by his bed and touched him to get his attention.

"Harl."

He looked at me sharply, sensing something important. I touched his chest and said it.

"They think they're going to have to replace your artificial valve."

His face showed pure comprehension. He sat straighter and looked at me, struggling for words that did not come. He pointed to his own chest and raised his eyebrows in a question. I answered yes, and his face crumpled in horror.

Did he understand me? He must have understood me. Neil, one of Dr. Friedman's P.A.s, came in shortly after and told him again. He sat up against the pillows trying to write notes, trying to ask questions, the strain on his face agonizing. Neil could not make sense of the notes and drew a picture of a heart, pointing to the valve that was to be replaced. Harl nodded with a look of understanding. When Neil left he cried.

I had meant to get home early this night, where my children who had never gotten along with Harl waited subdued and guilty and needing reassurance. They would have to wait awhile longer; to leave was out of the question now. I called and talked to David, seventeen and my oldest, telling him what had happened. Cathryn was sleeping; Steve was in his room.

Just since the stroke David had a new manner, very adult, very solicitous. He said he would tell Steve and Cathryn. I was not to worry, they would be fine.

Harl started crying again as soon as I came back in. I pulled down the bars on his bed and sat next to him, nestling into the familiar curve of his cheek and neck. He was so thin; in just these two weeks he had wasted to a skeleton of himself. How could he survive an open heart surgery?

He stopped crying and put an arm around me, from time to time patting or squeezing my shoulder. Each time I did the same to him, as the world outside his window went completely dark.

* * *

In the middle of his Sunday night dinner Harl's eyes suddenly fixed on the spoon in his hand. He looked transfixed; he said faintly but audibly, "Poon."

Then, very carefully, "Poon. Poon. Poon."

He did not think to look at me and rejoice. He was mesmerized, all his attention on the miracle of word and object. He said it until his voice grew so faint that he could not say it anymore. "Poon. Poon. Poon. Poon. Poon."

* * *

Five years ago I had waited with Harl's family in this same surgical waiting room through his first heart surgery. There were the same magazines, battered *Readers Digests*, an ancient *Women's Day* with a cover promising the newest makeup tricks. There were the same vinyl-seated wooden chairs, the same stale smell of cigarettes.

That first time I had been caught off guard, unprepared for my own feelings. A nurse came out regularly and told us Harl was doing well, everything was on schedule, he was off the respirator right on time....But a man was waiting with us that whole day whose wife was not doing well. Each time the nurse had to turn to him and say, "I'm sorry, your wife is having problems, we can't get her off the respirator...."

And when after many hours the nurse came and told us it was over and Harl was all right and we could go see him in Recovery, she had to turn and say to the man, "I'm very sorry, the doctor is coming to talk to you...." And the doctor came and said, "I'm very sorry, your wife died a few minutes ago."

I thought then how cruel it was for that man to keep hearing our good reports and think what he would give to hear those things himself. And I thought too that the day would come when I would be the one in his position, a day when Harl's heart would finally give out and a doctor would say to me, "I'm very sorry...."

This could not be that time, not quite so soon. From my spot in that dingy waiting room I pitted myself against fate, made my bargains. I would cope with the stroke, I would love him anyway, I wanted only for him not to die. Impossible not to feel when our own emotions are so strong that they must have power, must demand attention. Not thy will but mine be done.

Impossible not to feel that power, even when experience has taught us how pitifully unreal it is. I had once got up at five-thirty every morning and walked in darkness to six o'clock Mass, where I received Communion and when the others were gone--the others all old and poor, among them my pigtailed freshness must have made a shocking contrast--when the others were gone and I was alone in that vast church, I dropped pennies into an offering box and lit a red candle, for my mother who was sick. I was twelve and knelt in front of the candle rack and prayed, and in that awesome empty church I felt the certainty of my connection to the powers that decided everything, and knew she could not die.

A nurse came and said, "He is off the respirator. He came through it fine; you can go see him."

* * *

He lay in shackles, his eyes demented. It was two days since the surgery; the nurses called this I.C.U. psychosis and said it always passed quickly back in a patient room. The I.C.U. was disorienting with its lights and bells and no difference between day and night. And for Harl there was also his inability to speak, and the confusion of his own mangled brain.

It was too much; he had snapped.

I could not stand the restraints; I kept asking to have them removed. But he wanted to pull the respirator tube out of his throat, and he rolled his left hand into a fist and tried to slug anyone who came near him. He did not know me; he looked at me as if he hated me.

The nurses said *always*, but I knew always really means usually. Post-partum depressions "always" pass too, but some women stay in them forever and go to mental hospitals. For this to happen to Harl at the same time that his mind was shattered by its loss of words, and his ability to talk taken from him: wouldn't that make recovery less likely?

It was not passing all that quickly, even back in the patient room. I could no longer sit and stare at him when he gave me only those evil demented looks back. I roamed the hospital corridors, sat in the cafeteria and smoked, went to the door of his room and could not make myself go in. What was in there was not Harl.

* * *

Then one morning when I came in he looked at me and burst into tears, and I knew it was over.

Now he was crying all day, screwing up his face and starting to sob whenever anyone walked in. And the residents were talking about putting a feeding tube down his throat, because he was not eating enough to keep his weight up.

Sally the rehabilitation coordinator put a stop to that. She was the one who most often talked to me, her warmth and good spirits cheering me as nothing else did. She stood all the residents down, facing them with their charts and stethoscopes and serious abstracted expressions. She said coaxingly and pityingly, "You can't take a man who is depressed like that and put a tube down his throat. Give him more time; we'll get him to eat."

So Dr. Friedman wrote orders for him to be allowed a glass of wine with his dinners, and at each meal I stood by him, wheedling him into one more bite of egg or potatoes, one more spoonful of pudding. He resisted; his expression said food made him ill, and he did not understand the reason to keep eating. But his weight hovered where it was, and each day Sally and I exchanged looks of secret triumph.

* * *

They had added an antidepressant to his medications, but I thought it was more the beginnings of physical improvement that restored his spirits. Since the surgery he was no longer sick with the heart infection. And he could turn his hand now, and lift his leg.

Patty worked with him while I watched in the physical therapy lab, having him press his foot against her hand as he sat in his wheelchair. Patty was big and blond and cheerful, built like a tank and as inexorable. She had certainly chosen the right occupation.

She planted herself in front of the wheelchair, took Harl's hands and said unexpectedly, "Now stand up."

He still had the bewildered look of one who does not understand what has happened, or is happening. He seemed to follow orders as much out of this bewilderment as anything else, assuming that others understood what he did not and that he should do as they said.

When Patty said, "Stand up," he concentrated but did not hesitate. Balancing carefully, he came to his feet.

Patty produced a cane and said, "Now walk." Harl made an exclamation of astonishment, but there was humor in it. Patty's non-stop pressure and his helpless acquiescence had become a joke between them.

He took the cane, Patty poising her hands on either side of him for safety. He was still a bare skeleton of himself, shoulders gaunt, pants held baggily up by a belt that threatened to slide down over his vanished stomach. Patty could catch someone three times his size. She told him to move the left leg first; the right followed reflexively and he was walking.

My eyes misted: tears of joy, though of course I knew there is no such thing as tears of joy. We weep over something happy because it reminds us of something sad. These "tears of joy" were my unshed tears from the time I had thought Harl might be forever in a wheelchair.

He was concentrating on walking and missed my reaction. He went a few feet and back, thrilled now, beaming at me to share it. When he sat again he raised his hands to clap, left coming down over sluggish half-paralyzed right, for joy.

* * *

Carolyn had been coming in for speech therapy even when Harl could not make a sound, then having him just make movements with his tongue and lips. Now as his voice returned she began working on simple words and single sounds: "hi" and "bye," "m" and "b."

Harl would be exhausted in fifteen minutes, but he never asked to quit. I brimmed with optimism now, because his spirits were back up and because everyone had been reminding me of Patricia Neal's remarkable recovery from a stroke. If Harl worked this hard, surely he would be rewarded with recovery too.

Recently he had been wheeling himself up and down the hallways; once he had gone onto a sun porch and transferred himself to a lawn chair by the time a nurse found him. She laughed telling me about it: "He's just a really independent guy, and he needs to get out of that room."

But today something bad had happened. He talked in an unintelligible stream of gibberish, his left arm gesturing dramatically around himself and the room, very upset. And he would not go out.

The head nurse thought the morning nurse might have told him not to go out. "She was mad at him because he was having diarrhea; she was really mean to him."

I looked at her, speechless. Why had someone been allowed to be mean to him?

She said to Harl, "Did someone tell you you have to stay in your room?"

He screwed his face up, as if to say she was not making sense.

She said, "Harl, you *don't* have to stay in your room."

But he kept on looking at her the same way, and he looked at me the same way when I tried to tell him again. The speech therapists were finding that when tested without any nonverbal cues, his understanding was no better than would be expected from random guessing.

Yet there was the night when I had told him about the surgery, and he cried. Or Patty saying, "Stand up," and he at once stood up. Even in the ambulance when the attendant had said to blink his eyes twice for "no," and he did.

Or recently the times I wrote him notes saying, "I love you," and he smiled and promptly wrote back, "I love you!"

Those times of course there had been nonverbal cues, but usually there are nonverbal cues. He was extraordinarily intuitive too; the nurses had noticed that. He was understanding a lot.

I told him what I thought would cheer him up, sitting in front of him and putting a hopeful hand on his. "Dr. Friedman says I can take you out to dinner on Friday. Do you want to do that?"

He went motionless, and said his first sentence. The sounds were not intelligible, but the sense came through in the rhythm of the words: "I would *love* to do that."

In the hallway by the nursing station I confirmed the dinner pass with Neil. Harl still would not come out of his room but sat in his wheelchair just in the doorway, his skinny legs poking out pathetically from beneath his blue gown. His face was still a little crooked, and he watched us with a look of such desire that I was reminded, not disparagingly, of a dog hoping to go along on a family trip. Will he be allowed in the car or not? Those who can talk make the decisions. Powerless, he trembles with his hope.

Neil too saw that look, and called from across the station, "Harl is going out to dinner!" He wanted to dilute that intensity, stop that expression unendurable on a human face.

But it did not stop until I went back to him, and touched his hands, and smiled happiness as I told him we were going.

Each day Harl communicated through gestures, holding up his fingers, that he wanted to know how many days until we were going out to dinner. He kept careful track, showing each day on his fingers how many days were left.

That evening the nurses had him extra carefully groomed, dressed in his nicest clothes, his hair freshly washed and combed. He had gestured by moving his left hand as if putting on a jacket, and then as if stroking lapels, that he wanted me to bring him one of his sports jackets to wear.

A nurse thought to tell me he could have more than his usual one glass of wine. She whispered, as if conspiratorially. "What the heck, let him have two."

He waved goodbye as I pushed him to the elevator.

I was taking him to the Normandy, the best wheelchair accessible restaurant I could find in a reasonable distance from the hospital. Once I had not been able to name a restaurant; now I could choose among the best in the city for food and atmosphere and even wheelchair accessibility.

Harl stared out the car windows at the city sights as if he could never get enough of them. Waiters came outside and carried him in his wheelchair up the steps to the restaurant. Dapper in his jacket, he was able to read a menu and decide what he wanted. He read the wine list too, and chose the wine for both of us.

He even tried to place his own order with the waitress. His sounds were the sounds of a baby's babbling, bringing on in me the horror that was never far below the surface. But the waitress handled this as if it happened every day, just asking him to point to the items on the menu.

If Harl would be this way, perhaps we could be happy?

Everyone thought I was his daughter, because I loved him too obviously not to be someone close, but already it was incomprehensible that this pretty younger woman could be his lover. They could not know my memory of asking my stepmother for a bandaid for a blister on my heel, and having her say no. They could not know what this man had been to me, Harl who made the sun come up.

He sipped his wine, dark against the candles and white linen. I kept touching him to believe him, his arm, his fragile shoulder. Sometimes even touching should not be believing. On this night of so much happiness, I could not have imagined how far apart we really were.

The nurses teased him as they helped him back into bed, about what he had had to eat and drink. He tried to tell them by shaping his hands in the form of the small steak filets, then holding up two fingers to show there had been two. I stood happily back and marvelled at him and at these women, their energy, their real caring for him. And his own warmth, his personality coming through even in the thick of all this, making him popular.

By the next day all the nurses on the floor were talking about Harl's two steak filets and two glasses of wine.

* * *

Now he would inexplicably get the idea we were going out to dinner again when we were not. I would find him waiting expectantly, his hair carefully combed, becoming furious if we could not go. I sat trying to explain, saying we would go another time, we had to have a pass.

He did not understand. He seemed to think I had the power to take him out any time I wanted, that it was my decision. I wanted so much for him not to be disappointed that sometimes I succeeded in getting a doctor contacted and the pass authorized. But this was not always possible, and on nights we could not go, he could not be mollified.

His demanding began to cast a pall over the dinners out even when we did go. We never had another as happy as the first.

* * *

His children had come from New York to visit, Cindy and Fredd, bringing along Cindy's three-year-old. Neil gave us a weekend pass for an afternoon at home.

By now it was late August, in Evergreen neither too hot nor cold, perfect. We picnicked on the deck, Cindy and Fredd and I making conversation.

Would these two be able to make the role changes that Harl's calamity required? None of us had the knack of it yet. Fredd looked at Harl with his usual wistful greedy look of unfinished business; Cindy had brought the baby along in obvious anticipation that Harl would fuss over him and be proud of her. Harl did not have that in him now. He did not pay even perfunctory attention to the baby, seeming if anything disoriented by his activity.

Harl could not lavish parental attention on either his

children or his grandchild anymore...or on me, on anyone.

He stared around him, eyes lingering on the mountains, moving slowly over our yard. None of us could understand a word he said. My children fled, all teenagers now with plenty to distract them from this.

I could not have him at home and not take him to bed with me. After dinner I said with attempted discretion, "Harl must be tired. Let's all have a nap."

Alone in our room I helped him off with his clothes. He watched uncertainly as I came to lie against him, wrapped my arms around his scarred skinny chest. His eyes were still uncertain but bright with interest; I slid a hand inside his shorts. And then we were making love.

If this was still there for us, couldn't we be happy?

* * *

The Friday night of our next dinner pass, Harl seemed somehow to have gotten the idea he was actually being discharged and going home. When he realized I was driving back toward the hospital, he started shouting at me, a non-stop unintelligible stream of words.

He must be confronted eventually, and anyway I never could tolerate his being angry at me. I shouted back: "You don't make me feel much like doing nice things for you!"

Back in his room he sat in abject depression, saying nothing. I had no idea what to do.

I tried. "Harl, don't you know you have to come back here?"

He answered, the sense again coming through in the rhythm of the words, "Just go away."

I went to the coffee shop, smoked and wondered how in

the world I or anyone could ever manage him at home.

The other side of our love story: We had been fighting ever since living together, about my laxness with the children, my inconsistency....

How unfair he was to me, how unreasonable in his demands. He had always been stubborn, always thought he was right, never listened to me. I pulled rumpled kleenexes from my purse and wept tears of self-pity, not only for tonight but for all our previous life together.

By Sunday I was resiliently back, coming in cheerfully to where he waited in his wheelchair, to take him for another afternoon at home. My mind ran to the dinner I would cook, the warm fall day for sitting on our deck, then having him in bed with me again....

This time I had come up with the idea of making sure ahead of time that he understood the limits of the outing. He seemed to understand notes better than speech, so I wrote a note saying, "You will have to come back to the hospital tonight."

He replied:

> Mine back to Bonnie
> a short time later
>
> I don't want to go
> Evergeen = with Tonight
> if there is no possible
> of Evergreen green.
> The Evergeen under-
> standing under any
> evergreen before of as
> now
> even ~~now~~ of such
> understanding of any
> such cost!

Why was there that odd formality to his communications, as in "Mine back to Bonnie a short time later"? The struggle to organize his thoughts seemed to produce a sort of over-organization; the lack of readily available words caused him to use more obscure and formal words. Or perhaps this was an effect of the apraxia, the difficulty in initiating words. Difficulty initiating made him rely on formally structured initiations, to get going.

In this note though the meaning did at least come through. He blamed me for keeping him in the hospital and was refusing to go to Evergreen if he could not stay.

I turned on my heel and left. He sat rigid with anger, his face set, not minding my going.

* * *

Could discharge really be coming up? I almost could not believe it. Here in the hospital there were scores of people to meet Harl's needs. How could he manage with only me? How could I manage him? We lived alone up there in the mountains; what would I do if I could not control him? He would take off alone walking on mountain roads, or grab his car keys and drive off somewhere when he was not supposed to....

There was a discharge conference. Harl sat next to me in his wheelchair, seeming to understand some but clearly not all of what was being said. Carolyn was there, and Sally, and someone from the home health agency that would be providing Harl's therapists and visiting nurses. We discussed the arrangements I had already made: an extra railing on the stairs, grab bars for the bathroom. I had also placed an ad for an attendant, whom I planned to find and hire while taking my own vacation to get Harl settled.

A nurse was to visit three times a week. Speech

therapists and physical therapists would also visit, but one big question was how soon Harl could instead get to therapies in Denver. I envisioned him going daily to therapy as I went to work, for the better part of a day, this being his "thing to do" at this time. I thought he would be happier with this kind of schedule, and he gestured toward me and smiled and vocalized something to show he liked what I said.

The others demurred, saying he might be more tired than I realized. Sally suggested we might start with just two or three days of Denver therapies instead of five. That disturbed me; I was so eager for him to improve. Could we get home therapy the other two days?

Apparently not. Insurance companies took a hard line on providing home therapy to someone not completely homebound. We might get away with it for just the first couple of weeks, but after that they would probably not pay for both.

I brought up Harl's possible behavior problems, recounting his refusal to go to Evergreen with me that weekend. Carolyn, the speech therapist, was best at communicating with him and asked him about it. His gestures indicated he still believed I was somehow responsible for his having to stay in the hospital. Carolyn explained to him with her usual careful enunciation. "The doctors haven't let you go yet. That's not Bonnie's fault!"

He seemed to acquiesce, but I sensed he remained unconvinced.

Sally said to me, "*He* will have to have some limits set too."

She was reassuring me that it was all right to look out for myself too, not always to give him what he demanded. I needed that, but I needed so much more.

I did not know that swelling of the brain and other damage immediately following the stroke would cause Harl to forget even those things he initially understood. I had no idea he had forgotten he had the heart surgery and did not understand he had had a stroke. I did not know that many personality changes commonly follow a stroke.

And I knew nothing of what had gone on in Harl's mind during that psychotic episode.

Eventually he would be able to communicate it to me. First there had been a vivid hallucination of an adolescent girl--his eyes would widen as he described her--trying to seduce him. In the hallucination he was very conflicted because of me; sitting by me in our bed months later he would write for me that I was "wild" about it. Eventually in the hallucination he decided I was right, and gave up the girl.

It was only gradually over the next several months that Harl began to realize this could not have happened. And it was even longer before he was finally able to communicate about another hallucination, and find out that one had not happened.

In the second hallucination I told him I did not want him living with me anymore "since he was hurt." And I told him that during his hospitalization I was spending my nights with two different men, "a psychologist and a dentist."

So when I would return him to the hospital after taking him out to dinner, he thought I did so to go off and sleep with the psychologist or dentist. And in spite of all he had heard at the discharge conference, and all my talk to him of going home, he thought he was not going home.

He was discharged in late September, spiffy in his starched shirt and sports jacket, a day of sunshine on maple leaves. I buckled him in like the treasure he was and drove toward home and our new life thinking our relationship remained the same, that the only real change would be our method of communication. I did not know that he thought he was not going home, and that as he sat beside me looking out the window and saying, "Da," for either yes or no, he was looking to see where I would take him. I did not know that I did not know him.

CHAPTER FOUR

*We should not fear death. It is the possibility
of a life unlived that is tragic.*

---Leo Buscaglia

The first obstacle to Harl's homecoming was our house. It was frame, a modest mountain house and not at all conventional, but it was *us*.

Harl had sometimes been so moved by the view from our living room's picture window that he had to wipe his eyes. Standing by him, I asked him once if Psychology had an explanation for beauty, what evolutionary reason there could be for its power over us. He had not tried to answer, but only agreed: "It sure tugs at you."

No house could have been worse designed for handicapped access. I had wondered for a while at the hospital if we would even be able to go back there. The ground floor contained only a bath and my sons' bedrooms. One could not reach the main floor without climbing steep flights of stairs, either outside to the deck or inside from a narrow downstairs hallway. There were sharp turns in the downstairs hallway, first just inside the door and then another at the stairs. A wheelchair could not make the turns. Nor could a wheelchair get through the narrow door of our upstairs bathroom.

But Harl was walking with a cane and had been practicing stair climbing in physical therapy by the time he left the hospital. So the only modifications the house had needed had been the addition of the second railing to the inside stairs and grab bars to the bathtub. I did rent a wheelchair for distances.

He used the chair a lot at first, wheeling himself up and down the narrow hall between the living room and our bedroom. I listened for it, knowing my real terror at his homecoming had been not for practical difficulties but for the looming question no one could answer and that I would now have answered for me. *How was he going to feel?*

Perhaps not always so bad at first. The slight sound of the chair announced his presence, causing me always to turn and look. It was still shocking that he did not speak. But he had not collapsed into the anguish one might expect. I was there, eyes habitually on him, bolstering him with my own facade of cheer. Hating the hospital, he was happy with small luxuries of home: the beauty of the living room, the picture window, a snack brought to him as he watched television. His eyes sought me just as mine did him, turning to me at my every entrance, hanging on me with instinct that belied hallucination. I was there for him; he had to know it.

Indeed none of the behavior problems I feared had so far materialized. Was this the same man who had sat rigid with anger in his hospital room, refusing to come home with me for a visit? He seemed to be going an entirely different direction now, very gentle, very sensitive.

Our first task was to hire an attendant. I could have done this while Harl was hospitalized, but I wanted him involved. I talked to him about it as we sat in bed mornings drinking our coffee, never sure whether he understood my words, writing a lot of notes. What he wrote back would start out well enough to indicate he did understand, but quickly deteriorate into meaningless repetitions of words and letters.

The morning of the interviews Harl shaved and dressed

extra nicely, obviously understanding. He sat in his wheelchair as I talked to each of the three women who came, smiling and nodding, saying, "Da." One of them said as she left, "He is such a sweet man."

I would hear that word again many times. Harl had always been a kind man, might have been described as kindly. But sweet was new.

He knew without hesitation which woman he wanted to hire, the same one I did. So his values, his sense of people must be intact? Hope ballooned in me; this horror would pass and be like a bad dream after all. Harl would work hard in therapy and learn to talk again, and in a year or maybe two-- surely two--he would be himself.

Except that he would appreciate me more, for taking care of him. So he would stop criticizing me about the children, and we would never fight again.

We hired Melanie, who had recently moved from California and lived nearby. A part-time artist, she said the move was part of a decision to adopt a different lifestyle, more relaxed, less materialistic. Her questions about Harl were thoughtful; she seemed sensitive and unpretentious. I thought *godsend*; I liked her enormously.

Melanie would be starting full time in another week, when my two-week vacation was over. And before then she could come in for a few hours if I needed to be away.

How could I already be feeling I needed to be away, when it was still such a treasure to have Harl home? What I could not get used to was the silence, the not-talking. It hit me when the morning activities were over, coffee drunk and breakfast eaten, the children off to school. I went back and sat beside Harl in the bedroom or living room, and silence loomed around us like a living thing.

When the children were home they moved awkwardly

around Harl as he sat in the living room watching television, or at dinner in his wheelchair not saying a word. As a stepfamily we had been a disaster; it would be absurd to expect the children to starting dealing with Harl now. I would have to lead two separate lives, one with him and one with them.

From the time we started living together the children had rejected Harl by refusing to talk to him, almost refusing to speak to him. It was the one outward source of contention between Harl and me; he thought I could change them if I would only be more firm so that he was not the one always cast in the authority role, while I thought their perception of his influencing me to be "firm" was precisely why they hated him.

We had started seeing a family counselor a few months before the stroke, galvanized by a dinnertime blowup between Harl and Steve, ironically Harl's favorite. As if in mirror opposition to David's charismatic conventionality, Steve was quiet and agreeably offbeat, interested in music and photography and writing and art. Harl shared those interests, but he and Steve had never succeeded in having a conversation.

Harl had cooked a special dinner, pork chops in a plum sauce. After four years he had still not stopped hoping for some appreciation from the children, something besides their usual painfully polite, "This is really good, Harl," after which they would not direct a single comment to him.

Dinners had been grim ever since Harl started living with us, tension thick in the air as I struggled to make conversation with everyone as if nothing were wrong. I had a recurring impulse, never acted upon, to pick up my plate and walk out, leaving the four of them to hash it out for themselves.

Steve picked his pork chop up in his hand. Even I had never let him do that, but I would probably have confronted him humorously. Harl told him sharply to put it down. He did, but the children all looked sullenly at their plates. They would rather not have fancy dinners than have to put up with this.

Steve picked the pork chop up again. This time I might have let him; it was eaten closer to the bone, and we all did pick up bones. I did not think Steve was necessarily being defiant, but Harl took it personally. He threw down his fork and shouted: "If you want to be a complete slob, go ahead!"

My mind clicked in judgment. A therapist should know not to call names. Once I might have said so, but Harl had persuaded me I was "undercutting" him if I did not show a united front, so I never said anything in front of the children anymore.

Steve erupted: "You're a fucking asshole!" throwing down his own food and kicking back his chair. Harl sprang to his feet, blocking his path out, taunting him to fight: "You want to swing at me? Go ahead. Go ahead!" backing him into a corner, his chin thrust forward invitingly. Later Harl would insist that the fight was justified for him because Steve swung first, but he did not exactly give him a choice.

Steve of course swung. Harl was half his size and had a bad heart, but did know how to fight while Steve did not; he had him down in seconds.

Cathryn screamed at me to do something, and what indeed should I do? I thought the fight was at least as much Harl's fault as Steve's; my impulse was to pull them apart and tell them both to stop it. But I was completely confused by that "undercutting" business. And I knew what the children did not, that Harl was a very self-controlled person and would not do any real harm. Already he was pacing around Steve on the floor, jabbing at him as Steve tried to kick him, but not hurting him. He had landed just one blow before wrestling him down.

Harl had often predicted what he called an Oedipal showdown between himself and David, the importance to David as I understood it being to lose, and thereby be released to grow up. Was this that event, unexpectedly happening with Steve instead of David? Does a fifteen-year-old boy *want* his mother to save him from mysterious rites of initiation?

I fought back my own natural response and did nothing. So Cathryn screamed and ran to her room, and Steve finally released from the floor shouted that he would never eat dinner in this house again and ran to his room, and David who had been yelling at Harl all along to stop it now yelled that Harl better never try anything like that again with him *or* Steve because next time he would kill him, and ran to his room.

Harl gestured in magnificent disgust and slammed off to our room.

I had the odd thought that my children were at least better adjusted than my sisters and I had been. We had sat through years of gruesome step-family dinners, and none of us had ever erupted. Nor did I now. I began scraping half-eaten pork chops into the garbage, angry at Harl more than anything but feeling with my usual confusion that I should not be. Plum sauce stuck to the plates, a reminder of all Harl had hoped to give this family.

We sat a few weeks later in Bob--'s small office, the children sullen and grouped together, I next to Harl although at that moment I felt more like joining the children. I wanted Bob-- to be more definite with Harl, to let the children know he was not going to be just one more person who always took Harl's side. So far that seemed to be what happened, Harl and Bob-- the joint therapists here to fix up the children and me. Much later Bob-- would tell me he *always* saw me as the one most ready to work, but he had certainly not shown it so far.

It was Cathryn, now thirteen, who dared the system and

spoke. Bob-- had asked her why she didn't like Harl. Cathryn was dressed in bluejeans and her baggiest shirt; she had at this time a touch of junior high toughness. But she spoke sincerely and politely, with the clarity that was her special gift.

"Because he always thinks he's right, and he pouts."

"Pouts?"

Her eyes were resolute. In these last years they had gone from blue to hazel. Black lashed, they were so beautiful they made my heart ache.

"When he doesn't get his way. He pouts."

I did know what she meant. Harl called it getting his feelings out, but it came across as never letting up on anything.

I thought Harl would at least ask Cathryn what she meant, but he only made a helpless gesture, his face baffled and defeated. In his practice children had always liked him; he was known in his profession as "soft on kids." He did not understand.

That was our last session before the stroke.

I had been getting along better with the children ever since Harl's hospitalization; now in the shocking silence of this house I was increasingly seeking them out to talk to. But Harl and I needed adults to talk to; my next task had to be to get us some visitors.

We had been disappointed by our failure after moving in together to make friends as a couple. There was the fact of our both working long hours and living thirty miles from the city; there was the fact that most of the other people we knew also worked long hours, and perhaps in these hectic times of men and women both working, no one is socializing as much. But was it also something about Harl and me? We had an occasional couple come to dinner and spend an evening; Harl loved entertaining and was a wonderful host, and all of us seemed to have good times. Yet these visits never turned into friendships.

Someone said to me much later, "You and Harl always seemed as though you were complete without that." Perhaps true; perhaps indeed we did not try very hard. There was an occasional regret--"Why *don't* we socialize more?"--but for weeks and months at a time we hardly thought about it. What we wanted were our own Sunday mornings in bed together, our long hours of talking to each other.

So now when we needed company, when Harl would be seeing no one but his therapists and Melanie and me, and I thought already that I could not live through these long silent hours alone with him, I was having to turn not to close friends but to colleagues, friendly acquaintances, people who knew and thought highly of Harl but did not have a strong social history with him.

Yet they did care for him, so many of them coming to the hospital. I talked about it with Bob--, whom I had been seeing since the stroke by myself. Today Melanie had come to stay with Harl so I could keep my appointment.

Bob-- said, "Don't be surprised if not that many people come."

Startled, I wondered if he truly realized who Harl was. I said, "They had to keep them waiting in the halls at the hospital. Why would you think they wouldn't come?"

Bob-- said gently, "People are going to find it hard to see Harl this way. A lot of them may not want to do it."

Even if a lot of them didn't, that would still leave plenty who would. *Hundreds* of them pouring through the hospital. Mental health people. People who cared. Bob-- had to be wrong; I could find us ample social life if I worked at it.

I went home and called some people right then, couples who had been regular visitors at the hospital. Harl was home and ready to see people now; could they come for dinner this weekend or next?

Everyone declined; no one suggested another date.

I hated to ask people for anything; I was easily rejected. My hand gripped hard on the phone as I tried to think who else I could try. Because we had to have someone. The future stretched like an ice floe in front of me, jagged, desolate. I could not do this alone.

* * *

He had fallen, sudden as horror itself; flat on his back and then rolling down the carport, my scream following after. I was taking him to therapy; I had just moved ahead of him to unlock the car. Keys dropped from my hand as I went after him.

It would be a false alarm; he had to be all right. My arm around him, the texture of his jacket, his body so valuable, so valuable. Fetching his cane from the driveway, supporting him to the car. His limp was worse, the stroke-affected leg not moving right. Had he hurt it, did he hurt somewhere? He sat in the car and seemed confused, gesturing toward the leg yet saying no, no it did not hurt.

I drove with heart still pounding, recollection of how it happened slowing falling into place. I had been holding his hand. We came into the carport and saw that David had failed to put the trash toter out for pickup; trash pushed out the top and spilled over onto the carport floor. Harl made a familiar angry exclamation that said to me this was my fault, and I felt a familiar unexpressed defensive anger that said he expected too much of me, that I could not do all I had been doing for him and keep track of David's chore performance too.

Verbally unexpressed, but *I let go of his hand.*

Really I had let go only a moment sooner than I otherwise might have, but it had been enough to make the difference. Fear beat at my chest. He sat muddled and disheveled beside me, hopefully not too damaged this time, but what about future times? I had to stop my angers, had to be more careful, more careful....

He was not all right; he could not step on that leg. Because of pain? Yet he said it did not hurt. I took him to the hospital, heaving him into a wheelchair as he hobbled on his left leg and dragged the right. An X-ray showed nothing, no fracture, no explanation. The doctor on call tried to ask him where the trouble was, if it hurt somewhere, but he seemed less and less able to answer, saying yes one time and no another, making no sense at all. The doctor thought the problem must be pain, maybe a bruise of the hip. He said to go home and wait for it to get better.

I looked at him from a cavernous distance, his polite efficient face, *Go home and wait for it to get better.* He did not know what he was asking, what it was to get back in that car and go home alone with Harl.

Harl sat as I drove with his jaw set, staring bleakly ahead, saying nothing nothing nothing.

A day later he still could not walk.

I stumbled under his weight as I dragged him across the bathroom, asking *What is it, what is it?* The leg dragged uselessly behind him, and he could not say what it was.

He watched me from his wheelchair, his face rigid with fright as I began calling the home health agency. Their physical therapist had never shown up. The phone shook in my hand; my voice cracked as I said this was an emergency, they were supposed to have had a therapist here days ago, we needed one *now*.

She arrived a day later. I heard her steps on the deck and was at the door to meet her before she had time to knock: Effie, come to tell me what to do.

Harl still could not walk. Effie sat back on her heels, thoughtful. The only one of Harl's therapists who was not young, she was spry and vigorous and very experienced. She said, "When he fell, did he hit his head?"

I wasn't sure and Harl did not remember. But Effie was growing more sure of herself. "I think he must have hit his head. His brain was already swollen from the stroke, and when he hit it, that made it swell more. It may take some time for the swelling to go down, but he will walk again."

Until he did he was completely wheelchair bound, and our house nearly impossible. We would have to give up on therapies in Denver and use only the home health agency. Stairs were out of the question; what would happen if we had another fire and he had to get out?

But home therapy was probably better right now anyway, because Harl really was very tired. And what I most wanted *not* to have to do now was go back and face the people at the hospital. He had left them walking, discharged to my care. And what had become of him in just these two weeks of that?

* * *

Money at least was not the problem it might have been. Self-employment allowed me to earn a better salary than most women, at forty-eight thousand not enormous but enough that I could support our household by myself if need be. Harl and I had been fortunately too preoccupied with what we thought were more important things (my children, our work, our Sunday mornings in bed) to adopt the kind of lifestyle our combined incomes might have allowed. He had wanted to slow down and work less, and I only wanted to feel secure. The university would continue his salary for one quarter, then cut him to one-fourth salary for another quarter, then put him on unpaid leave if he still could not return. So between that and the loss of his private practice, he was going from more than sixty thousand a year to just a few hundred a month. Melanie alone was going to cost more than his whole Social Security benefit.

He could not meet his expenses without taking a loss to liquidate investments, unless I helped out. He drew a retainer salary from my company; I could continue that. And I told him I would pay half Melanie's salary too, since all of us benefited from her cleaning the house.

I had stumbled onto my occupation, private sector rehabilitation counseling, when Harl and I were dating, after a frighteningly long period when it seemed my degree in English had left me unemployable. I had taught English briefly on an assistantship and intended eventually to return to graduate school, but by the time I was divorced the baby boomers had caught up with me and college teaching jobs had dried up. I floundered, working odd jobs during the children's school hours, not wanting to teach high school and terrified of getting trapped in something clerical.

The job that came along was rehabilitation specialist, for a company that subcontracted from insurance companies to plan and coordinate vocational rehabilitation for persons injured in industrial accidents. The work was varied with much to learn; it had social value; it was not boring. I could even do a lot of it at home, going out to see clients and doctors and employers but making phone calls and writing reports at home when the children were out of school. They tumbled in and out of the room where I worked, excited for me: "Is that your *rehabilitation* report?"

Steve, then ten, drew a picture with my employer's name crayoned at the center in bright colored letters.

This was the job I brought myself to leave two years later, in the first year Harl and I lived together. I saw more opportunity for me on my own, and Harl said he would help support me if necessary through a period of getting my company started. Although that proved unnecessary--my salary soon doubled, then tripled--would I have dared leave the job of Steve's bright crayoned picture without that safety he provided me?

Harl had joined me in the company since, sharing office space where he saw his private patients and acted as our psychological consultant. He sat in on staff meetings, made decisions about psychiatric referrals and--his most enjoyable and important task--applied himself to keeping the company cohesive. Friday afternoons he set out Happy Hour drinks and snacks; joking that we all needed oral gratification to cope with our high stress levels, he kept a bowl of hard candies always available in his office.

He also did what he had never done at home, let everyone know explicitly that I was "boss" and never interfered at all with the way I worked. And he told me privately that he foresaw another role for himself down the road when, as must happen eventually, personnel problems came up. People handling was his specialty; he had managed the Colorado Division of Mental Health and could do a lot to help me manage this company.

So it was not unreasonable that I would use my company and my good salary to help Harl now. I had those things partly because of him; I thought as I waved to Melanie in the window and backed down the driveway for my first day back at work that now I could give him back something for all he had given me.

* * *

5:30 p.m. I came up the stairs carrying my briefcase, my eyes already seeking Harl. Always there was this fevered need to see him, to measure how he was, what he felt today. Usually he would be there on the sofa as I topped the stairs, his face lighting up to see me. He would say, "Hi!" Or rather, "I!," as he could not say the "h."

Today I had caught Effie's visit. Effie was immensely entertaining and kept Harl working. It was two months since his fall and he had only recently started walking again. I was so happy to see him walk that I would never have cared how well or badly he did it, but Effie razzed him without mercy, emphatic that he could learn to walk with no limp if he would work at it. No matter how well he did, she would remind him that he could still do better.

I was envious of Melanie and Effie for seeing more of Harl today than I had. My suit and heels in which I left the house this morning seemed out of place now. Melanie in her jeans sat comfortably on the floor. She had been with Harl all day, sat in on his speech therapy that morning. Melanie paid close attention to these therapies so she could help with the exercises between sessions. I did not want to do this myself; in fact I could not *bring* myself to be the one to hound Harl about his exercises, but I was jealous of her nevertheless.

They were having Harl walk back and forth across the room, keeping his arm down, carefully picking up instead of dragging his right foot. He picked it up only about half the time and did not seem to notice the difference when he dragged it. Effie kept him at it, and eventually he made a crossing that was almost perfect.

Then when Effie told him he could sit down, he promptly drew his arm up and hobbled to his chair in the classic gait of a stroke victim.

Effie rolled her eyes in exaggerated martyrdom. "A therapist's life is hard!"

Harl looked at her blankly. She practically screamed at him.

"You just walked clear across the room the way you're supposed to. Then you turn around and walk like this"--she got up and demonstrated, curling her arm up, dragging one foot behind her--"just to go two feet to your chair! *Why would you want to walk like that?*"

Stimulated by the vivid social interaction, Harl said with surprising clarity, "I don't!"

Melanie clapped in surprise. Harl laughed with her, but he had starting shifting his attention to me. This rapt attention he gave me was a subtly gratifying feature of his stroke. It seemed a sort of bonding, like an infant with its mother.

Effie left; I sat briefly in the dining room with Melanie to hear about Harl's day. She had brought paints and paper-mache so she and Harl could make masks, a project to entertain him. Gratitude spilled over in me; Melanie was so conscientious. They had made a perfect mold of Harl's face, but then he had refused to paint it. Though she did not say so, I sensed that Melanie was annoyed about that, feeling her effort rejected. I felt the same. With nothing else to do, I did not see why Harl should refuse to paint his mask.

The children were crazy about the mask and wanted to make more. Congregated in the kitchen as I cooked dinner, they asked why Harl would not paint it.

I answered as best I could, trying to defend him. "I don't know. Maybe he thought he couldn't."

That was inadequate, and they sensed it. They always did think Harl was a sourpuss. Closer to the truth would be that he did not consider this a task worth his effort. But tasks worth his effort were beyond his ability now. I had hopes for crafts as entertainment for him; he used to say he would like to dabble in pottery. Now he had his chance.

After dinner when the children had gone to their rooms I joined Harl in our room, sitting up against the chairback cushions we used for reading. Only now he did not read, just sat and watched me read. His reading had at first seemed intact, but it was not. The problem appeared to be with short-term memory; he could read, but he could not remember what he had just read.

What was left for a man like Harl if he could not even read?

I showed him my book, which a friend had given me: *Pat and Roald* by Barry Farrell, the story of Patricia Neal's recovery from her stroke. He looked interested at first, read the blurb on the cover--"...the story of Patricia Neal's extraordinary recovery from a massive series of strokes, and of her triumphant return to the acting career she feared she had lost forever"--and started to cry. But then he handed the book back to me, with a gesture saying he did not want to read it.

So I read as he watched me, and my heart began to sink.

I had been pinning my hopes on the Patricia Neal story, thinking that if Patricia Neal had recovered as she did, so could Harl. Now I was finding that her stroke had not even affected the actual speech centers in her brain; she was talking intelligibly three months later:

"I left Hollywood because I'd been in love and it had...not worked. Do you know who it was I was in love with? Gary Coo*pah*--that's right. Anyway, I thought that if I went to New York I'd get my life back like it was. And it worked because I met Papa--Roald!"

Whereas Harl at four months had just written me this note:

When the nearby world get to a shape which up to peaceful existence, will it be possible for one to live the small small apartment with then then charged with threw they they they hard a little harder?

Harl's tongue was affected too; worse even than not being able to find words was not being able to pronounce words. He sat by me in the cotton robe someone had sent him in the hospital, his right hand curled on the blanket like a broken bird, watching me. Watching me, and doing nothing else.

He was not going to recover like Patricia Neal.

Eventually I laid the book down and turned over and put my arms around him. What I remembered then was not the glorious story of Patricia Neal, nor anything from my own background in rehabilitation that everyone thought would be so helpful to me, but a passage from George Orwell, *1984*, that I had read in high school: something about the impulse to comfort, the reaching of an arm around a loved one, however futile to restore to him what has been lost--that nevertheless, where that impulse remains, a human being is not destroyed.

* * *

Christmas was coming up. I spent recklessly, both on the children and on Harl. Packages covered the floor for three feet around the tree, and went at least two feet high. I baked; I bought eggnog and chocolate covered cherries; I kept a fire going in the fireplace every night and weekend.

It was symbolic, that this place was still a home, that my own love and energy could make it still a home.

An ache in me would not go away. It was almost five months since the stroke, three since Harl had been home. I still rushed home every day with that fevered need to see him, yet it was terrible once I got here. Harl was not only silent but wooden; I could brighten him up for short times, but he always lapsed into that wooden lethargy again. I was beginning to grasp that brain damage was affecting more than just his speech.

Weekends were worse, because longer; I wandered about aimless and lonely, Harl glued to the television. For the first time in my life I had become interested in cooking, because it was something I could do and also because it was something he could share with me, in the choosing of the recipes. Saturday mornings we sat with cookbooks scattered around the bed, reading recipes and showing them to each other. Harl could read well enough for that and showed in his choices his old keen sense for cooking. But he steadfastly refused to try to cook himself, always gesturing toward his crippled right arm to indicate that he could not do it.

Concrete thinking.

When those mornings were over, the grueling lonely hours began.

A Saturday or Sunday afternoon, and he sat as always watching television in the living room. We had a smaller black and white television in our room, but to use the nice one Harl had to be right in the middle of the family pathways. Except for David who occasionally wanted to watch a different game, which I would tell him to watch in our room, the children completely relinquished the television to Harl, with no complaint. They relinquished the whole living room to him, scattered to their rooms as soon as he came in. He was so concrete, and so accustomed to his right to the television, that he would limp in and change a channel right in the middle of a program.

Harl saw David go into our room and motioned with outrage for me to do something. He had always been adamant that the children not be allowed in our room.

I explained. "He wanted to watch the game on another

channel. You were watching this one. I said he could watch it on ours."

He indignantly said something I could not understand, finally writing it with a flourish and staring at me with intense anxiety as I read it.

"My wallet!"

In the early months of our living together Harl had pointedly started putting his wallet in a drawer at night, because he did not trust David not to steal from it. Though David had never in fact stolen from it, Harl thought he had seen evidence that someone went through our things when we were away. It was not anything I would have noticed, but then I was unobservant. I did not think David stole from my purse, but he had been troubled ever since his father's and my divorce years before and had done some shoplifting. I could not say with complete confidence that he would not steal from Harl.

That was when David was fourteen. He was eighteen now, and since Harl's stroke increasingly helpful to me. More to the point, Harl *always* monopolized the television.

I snapped back at him. "I'll *get* your wallet. But David wants to watch a game too, and I'm going to let him."

In five years of living with Harl I had never made so simple a self-assertion. With all our fighting about the children, I had never simply said, "This is what I am going to do."

And I was not comfortable with saying it now, because it suggested I respected him less. More important than anything, than his therapies even, was that Harl not be treated as less than a whole person. I especially could not do that to him; the cheery little hospital pamphlets could say what they wanted about coping with strokes (they talked only about the patient's "frustration"; they never mentioned his grief), but I knew by now that whether Harl even wanted to live or not depended on me.

The other times, the times he was still himself: Christmas day when I opened the gifts he had picked out in a catalog and asked Melanie to order, items clearly of his choosing, showing his unerring eye for style and for me. He watched as I tried on a stunning open-shouldered sweater, beaming his old delight, lifting his hands in the air to clap.

And that night he wrote:

Bonnie, I am glad of the way the way the bag of Christmas! You bring off so many hurrahs! I hardly know the hand off claps!

CHAPTER FIVE

'I am,' I said.

--Neil Diamond

Melanie was growing exasperated with Harl's unwillingness to exercise. She said with a scowl one January day that this morning he had even lied about it, claiming to have done the exercises while she was downstairs washing clothes.

That was too absurd to consider. He could not switch his mind easily from one thing to another; he could not have come up with a thought like, "Now I will do my exercises."

But he never lied either, or at least never had before, which was what I said. Melanie was increasingly less tolerant of Harl than I was; I kept finding myself defending him. "Harl just isn't much of a liar. Maybe he didn't understand you."

Melanie shrugged and turned away.

Sitting by Harl on the sofa, I tried to talk to him. Didn't he understand how important the exercise was?

He shrugged.

"What does that mean?" I pulled his pen and notepad from his pocket and handed them to him. In the months since his stroke I had bought dozens of these small notepads; they were a staple on my grocery list.

He wrote something to the effect that "it doesn't matter."

"Do you mean it doesn't help?"

He nodded vigorously, looking pleased that I understood. I could still engage his interest in almost any conversation, and I sensed that this interest was what would bring back what was possible of his speech.

I said, "But it does help. It's just slow. You remember Carolyn at the hospital?"

He looked puzzled for a moment, then lit up and nodded.

"Carolyn said you might even go back to teaching someday. But the only way to get better is to do the exercises."

His face clouded. He made several attempts at notes that I did not understand, then suddenly came through with one that was perfect:

"I don't believe a word you say about teaching?"

It was a fluke of the stroke that as bad as Harl's word choice sometimes was, he always got his punctuation right. So I knew he meant the question.

"That was what Carolyn said. But even if you don't teach"--by now I knew in my heart he was never going to teach again--"you can still learn to talk to me and other people. Doesn't that matter?"

He nodded but accompanied the nod with another shrug, which belied it.

Now I did not know if he meant to say he did not think the exercises helped or did not think they helped enough to be worth the effort. Was just talking to me not worth the effort? I tried again.

"Do you understand that the exercises are what will make you better?"

He nodded again, but with the same shrug. I realized suddenly how common that shrug had become, and that it made me angry. He used it always at times like this when I was trying very hard for him; it was a put-off of my effort.

"Why do you shrug like that? Do you think the exercises will make you better or not?"

He wrote, "Not!" And by now he looked angry.

I touched his face, my anger dissolving in sorrow for him. "Harl, they will. And--" I faltered, staggered suddenly by the monumental truth of my words. "And I want you to talk to me again."

Something broke in him now; he began to cry. I held him and cried too, feeling his body racked with sobs. This was the part of him Melanie and the others did not reach. What they called "lack of motivation" was simple grief. How hard it must be for him to do anything with so much grief.

When he finished crying he gestured with both arms at the room around him. I understood he was talking about having to be here all day every day, not being able to get out and do anything.

I had an idea. "You can walk again now, and you're stronger. Do you think you might like to start going back to therapy in Denver, and maybe spend some time in the office with me?"

His smile spilled over me. He would *love* to do that.

So Melanie began dropping him off at the office after his therapies. And the hospital had also given us a device called a Lifeline that let him make an emergency phone call by hitting just one digit, to make it safer for him to spend some time alone. A portable switch attached to his belt, so that even if he fell or for some other reason could not get to the phone, he could still make the emergency call.

The hospital would call back, and if he did not answer, an ambulance would come.

Would he remember to use the Lifeline if he did have an emergency? Did he even really understand what this was?

Repeatedly he indicated he did, nodding and saying, "Eah," yes. He was excited the first morning I was to leave him a couple of hours alone, eyes bright, smiling to reassure me. He needed this independence; he did not like feeling he must always have someone with him.

And Melanie was getting tired of being with him, bored with the woodenness of him, frustrated by his lack of interest in his exercises. I understood better than I liked to admit; he was terrible to be with so much, terrible....

But I could not think that. I began instead to feel angry with Melanie, for not understanding that Harl's behavior was an effect of brain damage and not his fault.

For wearing out with him and making me fear she would leave when we still needed her so much.

For being free to leave when I was not.

I came up the stairs in the hurried way I always did after work, eyes seeking Harl. As soon as I saw him, I knew something was wrong.

His face showed not just his usual pleasure that I had come but relief, as if from some huge anxiety, as if he had been waiting for me for hours. He was gesturing to me at once, his lips already moving in a struggle to form words.

I dropped down on the sofa beside him and put my hands over his. I said, "Where's Melanie?"

He gestured in a frantic way that said that was what he wanted to tell me about; he said with a wave toward the door, "Dawn!"

"She *left*?"

He nodded, eyes wide, "Eah!"

She couldn't have, not without telling me. I said, "How long ago did she leave?"

He could not answer that, so I tried again. "Just a little while ago?"

He shook his head, and now with an eager look to show he had thought of a way to communicate it, he stretched his hands far apart.

"A *long* time ago?"

"Eah!"

Now his eyes hung on me, confused, anxious. I kept sensing in him things no one had told me about, in this case some lack of perspective, as if he had lost the ability to judge events in context. How bad a thing was this that had happened? Was it something I would want to do something about? What would I do?

I patted his hands, saying it was all right, I was home now, I would tell Melanie not to do that again. He watched me, uncertainly at first but then with the beginnings of relief. It was all right, Bonnie was here, Bonnie said it was all right.

Harl had written notes early in Melanie's employment with us telling me how much he liked her. Now I asked him what she did when she was there. He gestured with a pantomime of feather dusting that she went about cleaning the house.

A flamboyancy to that gesture, not something just minimally adequate but sweeping, graceful; and a comical facial expression to match. History of Psychology turned into a fairy tale; Harl had once told me good teaching took "a streak of ham."

I said, "But does Melanie sit down and talk to you? How much company does she keep you?"

He looked blank and replied that she didn't keep him any company. Now his eyes were anxious again. Was another bad thing happening? How bad was it?

I spoke to Melanie about the leaving, gently because I still hoped to keep her. "Harl needs to feel safe, he needs to know what's going to happen. And I need to know whether you're here or not."

Melanie said then that she was looking for another job.

*   *   *

A secretary said, " I think Harl is on the phone."

My heart stopped. He had not made a phone call before; I didn't know he could. I picked up the receiver, said, "Harl?"

He had rehearsed his words. First, "Heddo!"

Then, "Duh dady didn't dum."

It was the first day his new attendant was to drive him to therapy. I said, "The lady didn't come?"

"Eah!" He continued his carefully rehearsed words. "Ad I dote dow wat do do!"

I had developed a habit of repeating back whatever I understood of his speech. "And you don't know what to do?"

"Eah!"

He had been able to handle this, know when to call me and find the words to say.

I took over for him. "I'll call the Clinic and cancel your appointment. Don't worry. I'll get home early."

"Otay."

"Are you all right?"

"Eah."

I was reluctant to let him go. "Goodbye then?"

"Dood bye-bye!"

Only after I hung up did I realize how angry I was at the lady who didn't come.

We began trying to manage without an attendant, Harl riding down to the office with me on therapy days, staying home alone the others. At the office he thumbed through magazines or read books he had read before. His emotions were oddly out of control, what his therapists called *emotional lability*. He cried out loud over *The Life and Works of Sigmund Freud*.

I came into his office at noon to take him to lunch and therapy. A Senior Wheels van brought him back for me to drive home.

On the days he stayed home, he appeared to do nothing but watch television. Often I found him watching cartoons. He did not seem to change the channels, just sat by the hour watching whatever came on next.

My heart as I topped the stairs would sink suddenly, the idiocy of the cartoons bringing on the thought that most of the time I suppressed. This was my lover, the man with whom I was going to spend my life?

But always he lit up on seeing me; always he said that happy, "I!"

* * *

I had found him a counselor, an elderly speech pathologist who worked with stroke victims and their families. Someone who would attempt the impossible, psychotherapy with a patient who could not talk.

The three of us sat in Harl's office. Kathleen spoke in a way that reminded me vaguely of Harl before the stroke, a speech style at once articulate and oddly concrete, with a lot of visual imagery. A way of talking that could turn any story into a fairy tale. And she had a similar gift for precision, for getting right to the point of what she meant. And a similar careful thoughtfulness in what she said, a deliberateness that made one listen.

"Harl *remembers* what he used to be able to do. He remembers the lectures he gave"--she touched his arm--"don't you, Harl? And he sees himself now, and he doesn't want people telling him his attempts at speech are *good*. He remembers those lectures. He will not believe what he does now is good, and it will grieve him more to hear that. The better thing to say is, `Thank you for trying.'"

Harl was crying, taking off his glasses to wipe his eyes, nodding that she was right. He had started crying as soon as she mentioned the lectures. I reached to console him; Kathleen checked me by laying her hand on my arm. She said gently, "Let him cry."

I sat back. This was something I had already discussed with Bob--. Harl's misery made me so frantic that I put unreasonable pressure on him to act happy. He was never going to adjust if I did not let him feel what was appropriate, and express it.

But was he going to "adjust" anyway? I knew better than anyone the magnitude of what had happened to Harl, tortured myself with that knowledge constantly, but Kathleen's evoking of those lectures brought it home to me in a more vivid way. Less than a week before his stroke Harl had delivered a three-hour lecture without ever looking at a note. He had lectured countless times throughout his career and not used a note in twenty years. What hit me so forcefully now was not only his memory of those words rolling so effortlessly out of him, but his memory of the whole experience, the applause, the admiration.

The streak of ham, the love.

He might learn to speak well enough to function better socially, but he would never have that again. He pressed both fists to his eyes and wept for his loss.

Back in my office Kathleen talked more with me.

"I had misgivings as soon as I heard about this. Everyone knew Harl; I heard about him before you called me."

Why was that so gratifying? Had the lack of attention from his profession subtly affected my own sense of who Harl was, so that I would feel this warmth at hearing Kathleen reaffirm it for me now?

She went on. "When we talk about `adjustment,' we have to consider who the person was before. Those brilliant, high-achieving males are the ones who have the hardest time adjusting to a stroke. Perhaps it can't be done. Typically they will either get so angry that no one can live with them or so depressed that they are almost suicidal."

No one since Harl had spoken to me so directly. I had missed Harl's courage to admit reality, needing someone to help me look at this realistically. All that endless talk of "motivation" I heard from everyone else was a copout, a denial that something could happen (to them too, to anyone!) so horrible that a happy resolution was not possible.

I had tried to replace everything Harl had lost with love, but love was not everything. Harl wanted to be *himself*.

I told Kathleen he seemed to be taking the depression direction. He hardly ever seemed angry. Already he seemed to be conceiving of this as something too large for anger.

She asked, "Do you have a sexual relationship?"

We did, but it was drastically reduced. Knowing how important that was and hearing how easily Kathleen asked about it, I knew someone should have asked me this before. Dr. Friedman was a cardiologist, certainly not inclined to ask that kind of question. And even if Dr. Iminoff had not discontinued seeing Harl when he left the hospital, could anyone imagine his asking it?

I answered as accurately as I could, not pretending

concern only for Harl. "We do. Or he does anyway. It's better for him than me."

She nodded reflectively. It was good for Harl's emotional recovery that we had as much of a sex relationship as we did. I knew that and would not give it up, though it was not doing much for me. I had been resolved in those early months to reestablish as much sex as we could, satisfying to both of us. Idealistically, I had thought that anyone could have sex with someone in vigorous good health; to create satisfying lovemaking within Harl's limitations took *real* sexuality.

The one-sidedness of that effort doomed it to failure. Most devastating to me was that as if in unconscious protectiveness of his body, Harl withdrew from me not only sexually but even in holding and hugging and all physical contact. It was as if his muscles pulled inward and wrapped around himself instead of around me. He would suffer me to hug him, but he would not hug me back.

Anger rose in me; what was the use in such martyrdom? Harl's and my agreement did not prohibit other relationships. Our understanding, although neither of us had ever acted on it, was that we were both free to sleep with others as long as we did not lie about it.

I was barely into my forties. When I was not so shattered myself by Harl's stroke, I would seek sex somewhere else.

All that hung unspoken between Kathleen and me. She put it aside for another time. She said she would come back and see Harl again next week, next time preferably alone.

* * *

She came to my office after their second meeting to say

she did not have much hope for the counseling. Harl had to want to do it, and he did not.

My feelings were all so physical now, a literal sinking in my chest as I thought I would not after all have Kathleen to share this with me.

Kathleen looked out reflectively from under her white hair, speaking with that thoughtful deliberation. "There are a lot of ways that you and Harl are not typical of people who have to deal with this. Harl is only fifty-four, young to have had a stroke. And you are very young to be a stroke patient's support person. That may make it easier for you in some ways, but it makes it harder in others."

She was confirming what I knew already, that awareness of options made me more stressed. Had I been twenty years older, sixty-one instead of forty-one, I at least might not have had this panicky feeling that I was throwing my life away.

Though of course I could imagine another side to that, being sixty and seeing my life end this way. At my age I did have hope for a future that an older person could not.

I looked back at Kathleen and knew the real panic at the heart of me was in feeling my own youth slip away.

* * *

Kathleen had invited me to dinner. It was February, my first time out without Harl since his stroke in July. Kathleen sat opposite me talking knowledgeably about the food, smartly dressed, her white hair shimmering in the candlelight.

It took a setting like this--pampering, wine, dinner in a lovely restaurant--for her to soften what she had to tell me.

She told me over coffee, speaking with the care that lent

such force to everything she said. "Maybe I wish I didn't know what I know. But I have worked for twenty-six years with brain-damaged patients, and I have not seen a single case where this did not happen. I call it *loss of the ability to put another's needs ahead of one's own*; or perhaps I could call it *loss of altruism in the personality*."

Bluntly, I was going to have to take care of myself because Harl would never again put me ahead of himself.

Kathleen went on, gesturing in the candlelight. "Perhaps it is what we all want to do. We would all love always to put ourselves first. But as we grow up, we learn to block that. The brain-injured person loses that ability; he can no longer block it."

She had a story for illustration. She once had as a patient a recently married young woman whose husband was very much in love with her. The two had a special piece of "silliness" between them which had to do with drinking Cokes. When the husband brought his wife a Coke, she always gave it to him to take the first sip before she would drink it.

The wife was brain-injured in an automobile accident. When she came to and was able to sit up in bed at the hospital, the husband went to a soft drink machine down the hall and brought her a Pepsi. She opened it and promptly drank it down.

Stung, he thought, "Well, it was only a Pepsi." So he ran down the hall, found another soft drink machine and brought her a Coke.

She opened it and drank it down.

Kathleen's voice became emphatic. *"She had lost that ability to put another person first."*

The less than happy ending to this story was that although he stayed with her and continued to love her very much, this woman never did another thing for her husband that did not entail some advantage to herself. The husband had to teach himself to expect nothing from her.

One resists hearing such a thing. Relentless, Kathleen gave examples. If she and I should decide to see a play this evening after leaving the restaurant, Harl's reaction to my being late would not be, "Is she all right; is she hurt?" but more like, "Where is she when I need her!" Wasn't that true?

I knew it was.

Or if I was cold and Harl was cold too, he could sympathize with me for being cold. But if I was cold and he was not cold--if he should happen to be warm--wouldn't he expect me to turn the heat down?

I knew he would.

But why would anyone want to stay with someone who never put them first?

Kathleen said, "That is for you to decide."

CHAPTER SIX

Around the dear ruin each wish of my heart
Would entwine itself verdantly still.
---Ben Jonson

Harl and I sat together on our bed, a thaw of early spring outside the windows, I talking and he writing. He had begun to ask questions about the stroke.

> When did you sense my body being away from you?

I described again how it happened, finding him on the floor, pulling him up, calling the ambulance. He watched me with the most profound anxiety.

> *Something must have during the 4 days before the wake-up + the wrack-ups + now?*

    I gathered he was trying to ask about what happened next, the time in the hospital until he began to remember. I went through it again, the surgery, the therapy, his beginning to talk and walk. Stressing the positive, that he got better and was still getting better.
    He wrote:

> *Where is "date"?*

    He seemed to mean the date of the stroke. He could not

even place the event in time; he needed this kind of information to understand it. I told him July 25th; he wrote it back to me to make sure he had it right.

> Mon July 25

I asked him what he did remember. First he shook his head to say nothing. Then he wrote:

> My thoughts were returned to the hosp. & the deadening of its postesions. How the nurses cry — and the boldings hold on for just such a mass —

That must be what his memory was, a jumble of anguished sensory perceptions. No logic, no connections, just one day the capable man he remembered and the next the wreck he now found himself, with nothing in between.

Now suddenly he wrote on a different level, indicating some growing awareness of me.

> Bonnie, I am so depressed! You plan your game with so worthwhile a gent and then he disapears — and a nother comes on — and — and —

So he was not oblivious to my needs; he had been thinking about this from my point of view. And I was so wrapped up in him that even as I worked or drove, I kept hearing his speech patterns in the silences of my mind: the odd rhythms, all consonants coming out as d's. I knew the limping sound of his walk and would hear either that or some cadence of his speech in the dream moment of falling asleep. I was not even close to believing what Kathleen had told me, or at least not to acting on that belief.

Whatever acting on that belief would entail.

I told Harl I was more in love with him than ever and

would not leave him for someone else.
    He wrote:

> But look → here's the
> brand new '84 picture —
> I am now ~~that~~ picture
> and then you're in the new
> picture — the guy you're
> now sure you can keep
> around — the guy you're
> not sure you can ~~stand~~
> around — and the
> stand your in now &
> I wonder if ever ~~if gonna~~
> seen you way clear to
> say I say I've got it.

Meaning, "I've had it?" I told him no, I would never do that. And I meant it. He was there beside me, his body still warm and familiar, his face drawn with anxiety and hope. I held him, nestling into the soft spot under his cheekbone, promising my life away, telling him no, I would not leave him.

After a while I asked him if he had found any "good side" to the stroke. That was my own preoccupation, finding the silver linings: better relationships with my children, becoming more assertive myself, and then just the sheer piercing intensity of my own feelings, my own love for him.

Harl nodded at once, gestured between himself and me and wrote:

> *how I I'vd never feel this close before!*

I looked out our window at our melting yard, the water that ran in rivulets down from icicles on the sill, the firs with their still white branches dropping snow in soft clumps to the puddled ground. I thought that happiness is indeed perennial, and can occur under almost any circumstances.

* * *

Yet I would also feel myself incessantly pulling away from him, breaking the very intimacy I had thought would make the whole relationship worth the cost, because I was so weary of feeling his pain. Is it possible to be close to someone suffering as Harl was, and not suffer with him? I pulled from him and went back to him, went to him and pulled from him again. Closeness was quicksilver, lightning moments quickly suppressed. I held him and pressed my hands to his fragile shoulder blades, my cheek to the warm hollow of his, the scent of him a heat expanding in my chest; and then I left him in great bursts of efficiency, competent, getting things done, planning and scheming and daydreaming, my mind full of a hundred thousand things, anything but him.

* * *

Working at my desk, I always knew when it was two-thirty. Two-thirty was the time Harl finished with physical therapy and was picked up by the Senior Wheels van for return to the office. Because the van transported a number of persons, the trip was often long and roundabout. He would try to tell me about the people on the van and the places they had gone, his eyes widening with humor to show how far out of the way they had sometimes been, but this was something I could rarely understand. He was having experiences I did not know about; I found myself oddly jealous.

Four o'clock was usually his very latest time for reaching the office. How would he communicate if a van failed to pick him up, or took him to a wrong place? I did not *think* he would get off at a wrong place, but perhaps with his difficulties in understanding, someone could persuade him to. (He might think he was to wait there for another van? They were often late; how long would he wait?)

By four-thirty I could not work. The Senior Wheels office closed at five. I did not want to pester them for nothing, but if I did not call before five I would not be able to reach them. And what would I do if he never came?

One day the worst happened. The woman who answered when I called at four fifty-five told me the van had already returned, and there was no record of him. She was reassuring; she would try to reach the driver at home and call me back.

I called the hospital and reached Patty. She was shocked; he was picked up right on time. She would wait there until I called her back.

I paced the office, going repeatedly to the windows to stare out into the dark. Was Harl out there somewhere, lost, maybe cold, not knowing what to do? I knew how parents feel when they are missing a child: *God just let me know wherever in the world he is and I will go there.*

The phone rang; I flew to answer it. It was the Senior Wheels woman. She had not been able to reach the driver but would stay until she did. My voice broke as I thanked her.

At five-thirty there was the sound of the door opening and he came in, seeking me out immediately, collapsing into my arms. He struggled for words, too agitated to use his notepad. His van had been very full and only now got him here; it was a different van that had returned when I first called Senior Wheels.

His anxiety was over my concern, which he had realized I would have. So was Kathleen wrong, was he not really concerned only with himself? Was he perhaps not going to follow the typical pattern in that? I held him tight; surely I would not love him this much if he were as changed as Kathleen had told me he would be.

I called Senior Wheels again to let the woman know. Her own voice broke with relief. So did Patty's.

Then I bundled Harl into the car and took him home, where he would watch television and I would cook and talk to my children. Tomorrow I would go to work again, and wait for his van again.

* * *

I *dreamed.* Cathryn and I were alone in a place something like our Evergreen house, but bare of any furnishings. There had been a nuclear war; we waited at some distance for radiation to come. I had pills that we would use to kill ourselves. Otherwise our hair and teeth were going to fall out and we would die slow, horrible deaths. We knew the radiation was getting closer; we had started taking the pills.

There was not much feeling. Just waiting, and taking the pills. We sat together on a bare wood floor, waiting and occasionally taking a pill. My only real feeling was for Cathryn. I wanted to be sure she took the pills in time and was dead before the radiation came.

I could not think why I had this dream just now, but Bob-- did not find it so difficult. He thought Cathryn was a dream substitute for Harl, used to shield me from the real pain of what the dream was about.

"Whom are you really waiting with? Who has made your home bare, and who is it who is robbing you of your youth?"

At the "robbing of my youth" part, my heart made a skip

of panic. This had become my most compelling fear. Not only Harl, but because of him I too lived as if we were already eighty. No visitors, no sex, no conversation. My heart cried that I was too young for this. It was like having my hair and teeth fall out; I *could* not let my life be this reduced.

* * *

The worst memory of all, so burrowed into me I would lie in the nights years later and scream in my heart for release. Starting as things so cruelly do with something happy, a party invitation from a law firm for whom I sometimes worked. There was a moment, more than a moment, of thinking I might go alone: to meet men, by now I was always telling Bob-- I wanted to meet men. For what I dared think of only as a break, a fling, a release to help me keep on caring for Harl. Wasn't it what Kathleen had urged, that I look out more for myself?

But Harl too had no social life since the stroke, even less than I. I showed him the invitation, the other impulse fading as I saw his eyes light up. He gestured yes, he wanted to go.

I had not yet learned he would consent to virtually anything I suggested and that it was I who needed to screen social events for what he could or could not enjoy.

We changed clothes in our office after hours, he spiffy as always in starched shirt and jacket, I in the stunning open-shouldered sweater he had given me for Christmas. I steadied him on the ice in the dark, from the car to the building.

The other impulse not entirely gone: mostly I stayed by him, but surely I did not have to spend this and all future parties sitting silently by Harl? From time to time I left him with a drink by the hors d'oeuvres and went roaming, stopping with my own drink in hand to talk with the lawyers I knew: the men. Drunk on my own reflection under the soft light in the ladies' room, my sweater stunning and wouldn't anyone who saw Harl and me be curious about what was going on with me sexually? Didn't this whole scene in fact make me interesting?

What I did not know was how many people were here who had known Harl before, did not know of his stroke and would try to talk to him.

Either he must not speak at all, or he must speak in what he had by now learned was horrifying gibberish.

I returned to him so compulsively that I could intercept most of these exchanges and talk for him. Asking *did they know Harl had a stroke*. A lump rising in my throat then, how false the other was.

The party had been a mistake. He did not ask to leave but looked strained, his smile mechanical, his eyes distressed. I said, *Let's go*.

Yet I was stimulated, saying how much I enjoyed the party, asking as we reached the car if he had, too. He nodded yes, the expected response. But I thought to add, admitting reality, "Even though you couldn't talk right?" He burst into tears.

Appalled, I buckled his seatbelt and began the long drive home. As much as Harl had cried since the stroke, it had never been like this. This was new, the steady wrenching sobbing of one who has just realized the permanence of terrible loss. I had heard it before: lifetimes ago, when I was still married and my husband's mother learned her twenty-year-old daughter had been killed in a car wreck: the sound of a heart breaking, a weeping without crescendo, without hope.

He was witness to his own partial death. It was no less than that.

I could only listen and drive, navigating against funnels of snow that blew hard against the windshield and nearly obscured my vision. We were driving into a late winter storm, and those roads were icy.

*   *   *

Make it up to him. Whatever way you can.

He had been watching cartoons when I came home; I turned them off and gave him his mail. In it was an announcement of a Far East tour from the University of Texas Ex-Students Association.

I sat beside him as always when I came home, having a drink with him, my presence suddenly enlivening his world. First he showed me the tour packet for the pleasure of the pictures; then as a new thought struck him he raised his eyebrows for a question. "Doe?"

Anxiety; I could not really afford this. But travel was one of the things Harl had always most wanted to do. I paused, then smiled at him and said yes, rewarded by his look of radiant happiness. He clapped, and began right then to fill in the application.

By September he would be over a year post-stroke and surely walking and talking much better?   As we sat in bed that night the possibility of problems seemed to strike him for the first time. He had not stopped thinking about the trip all evening; now his happiness vanished and he asked, gesturing up and down his face to indicate the stroke, whether he might "mess up the trip."

The look of anxiety so abruptly replacing the radiance moved me to excessive reassurances. "No, you won't mess it up. You'll be better by then. And I can help you."

He looked away, staring across the room with a long internal look that was reminiscent of his old self. Harl had always considered and deliberated in that way, a methodical, purposeful life approach that contrasted my own impulsiveness and in former times had often grated on me. Now I treasured it in him, just as I did his continuing impeccable neatness: his watch and wallet laid carefully in their appointed spots in his top bureau drawer, his nails perfectly clipped, his person immaculate as ever. I had heard of stroke victims becoming personally slovenly; Harl's character went too deep for that.

After a few moments of that thoughtful considering look, he seemed to decide that I was right and did not worry about it again.

I on the other hand had committed to the trip on a moment's impulse and would have misgivings for months after. Anxiety woke me in the nights. Would I really be able to handle this?

By September he was not walking or talking much better than when we first signed up, but he was living for that tour. Night after night we sat up in bed and looked at pictures and talked (wrote notes) about it; during the days when I was gone he did the same. I had an uneasy suspicion that he was thinking of killing himself when it was over. The trip was perhaps to be his last good time, the thing he had always wanted to do before he died.

Kathleen told me she had never known of any stroke victims killing themselves, apparently because they cannot get organized enough to do it. I took comfort in that but still had the fear. Braced for Harl to bring it up, I had worked with

Bob-- on my response: that I would understand if that was his decision, but that for my part I wanted very much for him to live.

And that he should wait and see if he got better. Postponement is everything with a suicide.

By our departure day Harl was wild with excitement, up and dressed and tucking his passport into his pocket. Photographs would show Harl radiant: smiling from his wheelchair in a Japanese garden, or dwarfed by a gilded Buddha. Photographs of the two of us, snapped by an occasional thoughtful tour member, show me behind him looking perhaps not too much different from my usual picture look: dutiful, a hand on his shoulder, concerned in that moment mostly with how I am going to photograph. But something noncommittal in the eyes contrasts Harl's straight-forward happiness. It is a look that says *I know this is a wonderful thing that I am incredibly fortunate to be able to do, but perhaps people should not do such wonderful things when they are so raw with loss that it all rolls off of them.*

My look is shellshocked.

So many airports, all running together: Japan, Singapore, Hong Kong, Thailand. I pushed his wheelchair to our planes, and he stood and walked on. I followed, feeling each time a pang as he moved promptly into the window seat. He would then beam at me, having no notion what he had just done. Harl had loved introducing me to travel and in the past always gave me the window seats. Like the man whose wife no longer gave him the first sip of Coke, I wanted not the seat but the gesture. It was a loss.

He sat by our Hong Kong hotel window, studying tour literature as I napped. After a year of casting envious glances at his antidepressants as I shook them out for him each night, I had finally obtained my own prescription to help me through this trip. It must have been partly the antidepressants that were making me sleep this way, but I was afraid to stop taking them. I was terrified of how I might feel on this trip without them.

That my own internal landscape might collapse on me was always my deepest fear. Better to sleep like the dead every afternoon than to risk that happening.

It was Harl who was high on the trip, ready for every outing, wanting to miss nothing. One of the restaurants where we could use our dinner coupons was Hugo's, according to the travel literature and also to Harl, who retained the knowledge of the sophisticated man he had been, one of the best restaurants in the world. He gestured toward it in the pamphlet as he saw me beginning to wake up, smiling as he had been doing through all the months of planning, clapping his hands.

I tried to feel as I pushed the wheelchair out into the evening some sense of adventure. Cabs were waiting; our driver loaded the wheelchair into the trunk. We settled in and I told him to go to Hugo's.

He asked me where that was. Nonplussed, I wondered how I was supposed to know. This was supposed to be one of the most famous restaurants in the whole world. Didn't all the taxi drivers in Hong Kong know how to get there?

When I told him it was a restaurant, he said, "Ah!" and took off. Apparently he had remembered.

I had thought it was on our side of the channel, but he headed across the bridge into Kankoon. I watched him put ten dollars in the turnstile. Several of us had made this trip for shopping earlier in the day, and I heard some of the others say their drivers overcharged them for the turnstile, claiming to have put in twenty dollars rather than ten. Our driver had not done this to us, perhaps because he sympathized with Harl.

This one did. He also overcharged by at least four times for the trip itself. Harl could only sit helplessly waiting for him to bring around the wheelchair; I who once could not name a restaurant was halfway around the world having to handle this by myself.

I was always on the side of the underprivileged; I could sympathize with those who serviced rich American tourists. They knew we had the money to get here, and the amount of the overcharge was negligible in American dollars. But Harl was underprivileged in his own way too, and I was as lonely as I had ever been in my life and about to sit through one more silent dinner with him. I found myself nearly in tears, so angry that although I knew the only reasonable thing to do was pay, I did speak up.

"I saw you put ten dollars in that turnstile. And we came over this morning for less than half this much."

He shrugged angrily, demanding his money. Normally I tipped well for the handling of the wheelchair; since he had already ripped us off, I at least did not tip him. His tires squealed as he left us on the pavement, where we had to negotiate a short flight of stairs.

Harl was fortunately able to stand and walk up the stairs while I dragged the wheelchair up them backwards. Inside the hotel I was still trembling, brushing tears from my eyes as I struggled with my own obvious over-reaction. I did *not* blame struggling Hong Kong taxi drivers for taking some advantage of American tourists. My reaction was because Harl's calamity was so terrible for him, and being with him so hard for me. I wanted sympathy.

Hugo's was not here; we had been brought to the wrong place. A desk clerk told me Hugo's was back across the channel, just as I had thought.

Could our driver have done this on purpose, to get the

nice fare? It was hard to think that badly of anyone, but surely all the taxi drivers in Hong Kong knew where Hugo's was.

I started to push Harl back outside to get another taxi. Unexpectedly he stopped me, holding his hand out against my arm, trying to console me. He thought I was upset about the taxi money; he gave me a huge reassuring smile and pulled out his wallet to show me he had plenty of money.

The simplicity of that gesture made me really begin to cry. He patted my hand and gave me the warmest smile I had ever seen; Ben Kingsley as Gandhi.

I leaned down to lay my cheek for a few moments against his, then went on outside with new calm to find a taxi.

Dinner at Hugo's was of course wonderful, a haze of crystal and candles and three waiters standing around to serve us. Was such a dinner worth the silence in which we had to eat it?

Harl patted my hand repeatedly, smiled and gestured around us, wiped his eyes for joy.

* * *

We were back in Colorado sunshine, shopping for a car. This one was a five-year-old BMW, black with a cream interior, beautifully cared for. Harl limped around it, smiling, motioning to me to open the hood. Sun reflected off the hood and off Harl's hair, showing its first shades of gray.

We had taken the car for a test drive already. The owners waited by the driveway; Harl made his last inspection and motioned to me to talk to them. His face had a look of satisfaction that I had not seen there since his stroke.

He had passed a driving evaluation at Craig Hospital,

coming back and limping into my office with the papers in his hand to share that triumph with me. His smile then and now was his old smile, never a mouth smile only but the kind that moves the whole lower part of a face.

Hope was quick in me; I always thought that if Harl was happy, I could be too. I stood in the sunshine in the driveway making arrangements to come back and pick the car up on a weekday for an inspection. Harl stayed modestly behind me with a hand on the car's gleaming fender, smiling his own goodwill.

Three days later he had the car. I had some notes printed for him, Kathleen suggesting the language:

> I am Harl Young.
> I have had a stroke.
> Please wait and I will be able to
> tell you what I want.
>   THANK YOU.

And on the back, my name and phone numbers in case of emergency.

Now he could take himself to therapies, no longer spending afternoons in my office but driving home to sit on the deck or watch television, and light up and say, "I!" when I came in.

* * *

We were making what seemed it might be the beginnings of a new friendship, with Ray and Virginia, a couple who accepted our occasional invitations and even occasionally reciprocated. Tonight we were to meet them at a restaurant in Denver, but the weather was turning bad. I worked in the kitchen, listening to weather reports as I got the children's dinner ready. The highways weren't going to be bad, so we could still go. But the roads in Evergreen were treacherous, and I needed David to go to the grocery store for me.

My car was in the shop, and David's was an ancient Buick Skylark that was not safe on the ice. I walked to the living room and said to Harl, "I need David to go to the store, and his car isn't safe in the snow. Can he take yours?"

He looked at me and said flatly, "No." The look on his face conveyed that this was an outrageous request.

Who had spent a weekend taking him to look at cars? Or left work to take the car in for an inspection, or gone to the bank to arrange his financing? Who had set up the driving evaluation for him in the first place?

I sat down and got his attention to make sure he understood. I said carefully, "The shopping is for you as much as for anyone else. David and I always do your shopping for you. And his car doesn't have snow tires, it isn't *safe*."

He still said no, without even the courtesy of an argument, his manner indicating there was nothing to argue about. Kathleen was right; he could not care about any point of view but his own.

Sixteen months of taking care of him, and I had never once even been really cross with him. Now I began screaming: he was totally selfish, I was doing everything for him for nothing, I could not stand any more of this, I did not want to go out with him that night.

Harl followed me to our bedroom and watched in silence as I finally threw myself on the bed to cry. When I was through, he made his first and only response: had I really meant it about not wanting to go out that night?

None of the rest had mattered, only the part that immediately affected him. He was a monster.

Yet I did after all go out. That was what shocked Bob-- the most when I told him. He said he did not see how I could have done it.

I thought that over. "It was because of Ray and Virginia. I didn't want to cancel on them."

"But couldn't you have gone out with Ray and Virginia on another night? Didn't your own feelings matter, to you if not to Harl?"

Apparently not, if I could not get Harl to agree with them. I had really not wanted to go, and it had been a terrible evening. The weather could have been an excuse to cancel. And was it entirely because of Ray and Virginia that I went, or was it also that in spite of everything I had not wanted to disappoint Harl?

But Harl had deserved to be disappointed. That selfishness made him less than human; I could not live with it, and he could not be allowed to go on with it. He was relearning so much else; might not concern for another person be something that could also be relearned?

Bob-- said, "I don't know. You could talk to Kathleen about that. But I know this, he is not going to learn it unless you teach him."

* * *

Disaster is earthquakes, bombs, a lover felled unspeaking on the floor. But disaster can come quiet as a cat, or a ringing in an ear.

Cathryn said as we shelled shrimp at the sink, "Mom, you need to move to Denver. We should move."

I looked at her in surprise, fifteen and lovelier by the day, in her first year of high school. Living in Evergreen was isolating now; I had talked about moving off and on since Harl's stroke. But I had been reluctant to make the children change schools, and Cathryn at first had said she did not want to.

I said, "I thought you said you didn't want to move."

She said, "I didn't. But David and I have been talking about you, and we're worried about you. You need to move. I can handle it."

Was I that obvious? I had not really talked to the children much about Harl, not knowing what to say. I had meant to model for them appropriate behavior in a crisis, and appropriate commitment to a loved one. Strength. I had not known with what clarity they would see instead my inside suffering.

Saturdays while Harl watched television Cathryn and I drove to Denver to look at houses. She brought tapes to feed the deck: David Bowie, Junk Culture. I liked them; I liked being in a car with music playing better than anything, because the sound masked an increasingly annoying ringing in my left ear.

I complained of the ringing to Harl, plugging in a vaporizer as we went to bed at night. I always woke up in the nights; I might as well plan for it. The vaporizer would mask the ringing.

A little ringing in an ear was such a small thing next to Harl's problems that it seemed self-centered even to complain of it, but it was really terribly annoying. Harl would look at me and nod as if interested--he was interested in everything I said, he was so starved for words--but he never asked me about it on his own. Cathryn did; I told her I was going to see a doctor.

I had no hearing loss, so Dr. M-- did not think I had a tumor. He thought it was routine tinnitus that I would have to "learn to live with," but he scheduled me for a CAT scan just to be sure.

I would tell the story this way.

Making a joke of it.

I knew of course that I did not have a tumor. Nothing was ever wrong with me; if anything I hoped for a tumor because I assumed it could be removed and the ringing stopped, but I knew I would not have one.

So I had resolved to conquer this with mind control. I would find a hypnotist. If people could be hypnotized out of hearing things like horns blowing, why couldn't I be hypnotized out of hearing my ear ring? I would find a hypnotist, and in the meantime I would self-hypnotize myself. I would get my attention off it; I would make myself not hear that ringing.

That was my whole concentration as I lay in the CAT scanner and later as I sat through tests at the Denver Ear Institute, hooked to machines that rotated me and made clicking noises. I would not hear that ringing. I would not.

Right in the middle of one of the tests a nurse came in and stopped it. She said my doctor was there and wanted to talk to me. We were not going to finish the test.

I thought what a coincidence Dr. M-- should happen to be there just when I was being tested.

He took me into an office and sat next to me. He said he had reviewed the CAT scan and came over to talk to me about it.

I thought that was nice.

He said I did have a tumor, a large one.

I thought that was wonderful. It meant something could be done; I would have an operation to remove the tumor and the ringing would stop. I said, "Oh good! So you can stop this?"

He looked perhaps a bit disconcerted but went on. If we had caught the tumor when it was small, it could have been removed by an approach that did not damage the ear. Most people had symptoms long before I did; most would have been having all sorts of hearing and balance problems by the time a tumor got to the size of mine. Actually he had never seen such a large tumor with so few symptoms. It was so large that the more favorable approach was out of the question, because his concern now had to be saving the facial nerve. He would have to approach from behind the ear, destroying the whole inner workings of the ear on the way in, and even then he could not guarantee me an intact facial nerve. The left side of my face might be paralyzed.

I was still not comprehending. "Then how do you reconstruct the hearing?"

They could not reconstruct it. The outer ear would remain, but I would be completely deaf in it.

It was not possible. What if I just didn't have the surgery?

The tumor was already stuck to the brainstem and would keep growing. It would kill me eventually. Meanwhile my face would become paralyzed and I would lose my hearing anyway. We had to get it out quickly; the larger it grew, the more damage to the facial nerve. I could get another opinion if I wanted, but he had studied under the top person in this field and knew for certain anyone else would tell me the same thing.

I groped for other possibilities. What everyone expects: the near miss, the squeal of brakes, no of course the child is not hit; how could he be hit? Later you will hold that child and say with wonder, *It missed him by an inch*. But already this will seem the only possible outcome. So long do we live on the edge of disaster that we stop believing it can really happen.

So it would be now, the reprieve that had to come. Any moment this doctor would say, *Well, there is this one other possibility*....

Wasn't there then? Wasn't there anything that might save my ear?

No.

My world ended.

CHAPTER SEVEN

*There must be in the heart a faith so faithful
that it comes back even when it has been slain.*

--Rostand

I drove alone toward home, navigating the familiar highway. I would be handicapped, *hearing impaired.* I would have to ask people to speak up, say, *I can't hear you, I am hard of hearing.*

And I might be disfigured, my face grotesque. The beauty that was the sweet surprise of my adolescence gone, and without it would I ever have any love or sex again?

If I could never have another man again, would it be possible for me to be happy with Harl?

With Harl's stroke I had steadfastly refused popular blame-the-patient notions of illness as metaphor. I did not believe Harl had "chosen a sick role" or that his stroke expressed some underlying psychic reality. Mostly I agreed with Susan Sontag that those notions are based on little or no evidence; mostly I thought illness was *not* metaphor.

But maybe sometimes it was, and maybe this was one of those times. There was something spooky about my losing an ear as if in response to Harl's losing his speech...my *left* ear even, the one I most habitually turned to him, because of holding his crippled right hand. Did my ear grow sick from not hearing him talk?

Was this what Psychology called an *enmeshed* relationship?

And what was this feeling of *betrayal*? I had denied to myself that what I did for Harl was martyrdom, done with a martyr's expectation of reward. But why else should I feel betrayed? To lose my ear, that was my reward.

I told David first, pulling him into the kitchen where Harl could not hear. David would need to postpone a trip he had been planning to take with high school graduation money. Harl could not run the house or manage himself without me; much as he was going to hate it, he would need David. All of us would need David.

I did not think then that those few words I said to David in the kitchen that night would change him and his life forever. He was a young man, planning for college and well past the troubles of his early teens. But this was the first time his feelings for his family had been challenged by major responsibility. David take care of Harl? He would have to; there was no one else.

David said of course. Of course he would help, of course he did not mind postponing his trip. The stunned look in his eyes was for me, that this was happening to me.

I went back into the living room to tell Harl. Tears welled in his eyes; he had no words to answer me. By now I had numbed myself and did not cry with him. But when Cathryn cried on hearing it, I did. Harl cried all the time; there was a more moving depth to Cathryn's tears.

* * *

My sister Robin flew in for the surgery; Leslie would

come when she left. Instead of making us closer, the traumas of our family life had seemed to drive my sisters and me apart; as recently as Harl's stroke I had not even called them. I had not told anyone in my family about the stroke until months after it happened.

Since then Robin had been calling me; that renewed relationship was high on my list of silver linings.

Harl went about in a stupor, completely absorbed with me, dysfunctional without me. He had often had difficulty remembering my name, but now he suddenly began calling me "Mother." I could only think this was an emotional connection his mind was making, out of his fear of losing someone on whom he utterly depended.

Robin said I should see if he might be allowed to spend the night before the surgery in my hospital room with me, perhaps sleeping in the other bed.

It was not common practice, and it was taking some chance because no one could be sure how Harl would behave, but Dr. M-- consented. Kathleen had told me he was a good person.

Oh, and this was not just for Harl! No longer miserable looking and withdrawn, he sat by me in stroke-forced silence with all the warmth of his old personality wrapping around me. Everyone had been wonderful to me, Robin, Leslie, Kathleen, my children. But in this last night before I was to have my ear cut out and possibly my face ruined, it was Harl I wanted.

Kathleen had given me pre-surgery relaxation tapes; Harl listened to them with me, over and over. He held my hands, patted my shoulders, smiled comfortingly and watched me until I fell asleep. I had been crying every night, but I did not cry that night. When I woke Harl was there, already up and beside me.

Robin would tell me later that when she first saw me in Recovery, I was calling for him.

* * *

I spent two days in Intensive Care, hallucinating and throwing up. But my first thought on waking, and throughout that bizarre and unreal time, was that I could close my left eye. My face was not paralyzed; I had been spared that.

Back in my room, I lay limp with exhaustion. The nausea was past, but I was still violently dizzy. I knew the luxury of complete dependence, waiting passively for those who came to visit or care for me.

A glimmer of something, like a teenaged girl who wants a baby to love and care for, when what she really wants is someone to love and take care of her. This caretaker role of mine was hooking into something deep.

Dr. M-- fairly beamed with pride that he had saved my face. I watched him and listened to him and found it miraculous that a near stranger would have made such an effort for me. The tumor was so large that it was stuck to the brainstem and even the cerebellum; it had taken twelve hours, half again as long as estimated, to scrape it from there and to peel it meticulously off the facial nerve. He could have rushed it, damaged the nerve, and I would not have known the difference. But he had not.

Kathleen was so happy that she took the doctor flowers, finding him the next morning working in his garage. Why did she care that much about me? Why did anyone?

Harl was radiant, his whole face a smile. Robin told me about waiting through those twelve hours with him, and how changed he was when it was over and I was all right. The doctors were so concerned about him that they advised against letting him see me in Recovery. But the next day he took Robin to tour the D.U. campus, expansively happy, motioning to her all the right turns to get to the places he wanted her to see.

Later, with Leslie, he was driving and suddenly could not remember where or why. They pulled off the road and Leslie talked to him, telling him they were going to see Bonnie, that Bonnie was in the hospital. He would say, "*Bonnie* is in the hospital?" and she would say yes, remember, Bonnie is in the hospital....

Leslie asked Kathleen about it; Kathleen said it was probably entirely emotional.

* * *

At home I continued both in the weariness and in the strange pleasure of major body trauma. Too weak to do anything, I did not have to do anything.

Harl was totally interested in me, willing to spend hours lying beside me. Yet he had not made a single preparation for my homecoming. Leslie before she left had arranged for a home health aide. The aide spent most of the first day throwing out spoiled food from the refrigerator, putting clean sheets on my bed, cleaning the bathroom and shopping for food that I could eat. It had never occurred to Harl to do any of these practical things for me; his notion of caring for me was to lie beside me, to express love and sympathy.

Limp with exhaustion and relief, I did not have it in me to feel angry over his lack of practical assistance. That was a result of brain damage, not his fault. I would appreciate him for what he was. My children raced home after school to see me. Cathryn brought me snacks and water; Steve plucked the year's first crocuses from the snow and put them in a vase beside my bed.

Harl drove himself to therapy three mornings a week. The hours alone were treasures, Dixie bringing me eggs and toast and coffee, lying in that indescribable peace looking at my flowers or out the window at the sunshine on the snow.

Harl's homecomings were treasures too. He came always directly to our room, already pulling out his wallet to lay in its appointed spot in the bureau drawer, still radiant because I was alive and my face was not paralyzed. He would lie beside me the rest of the afternoon, happy to do nothing but be near me, until the five o'clock news came on. I drifted in and out of sleep; when I woke he was always there.

* * *

I had made an offer on a house in Denver's Washington Park area three days before my tumor was diagnosed. The closing was three weeks after my surgery. We moved at the end of April, seven weeks after the surgery.

Ray and Virginia helped us. I stumbled around packing and cleaning; Harl sat on the sofa and watched, packing only a few of his own belongings when I instructed him to. The same thing happened at the other end, with unpacking, except that now we did not have Ray and Virginia helping. My dizziness was still violent; I had to return to bed for several days.

In fact my balance compensation was not occurring on

schedule. Dr. M-- had predicted a part-time work return about three weeks after surgery. I could not work even after eight weeks, my dizziness becoming so violent that I would have to return home and lie down. And it was still impossible to do prolonged reading, which between reviewing counselor reports and researching my own court cases was seventy percent of my work. Dr. M-- said the reading difficulty was because there is some coordination between the eyes and the ears; my left eye was still not working correctly with the right.

He sent me for an ENG and Rotary Chair Test; both indicated I had not even begun to compensate. But he could not tell me why. He said slow compensation is expected in the elderly, but he had never seen this before in someone as young as I.

All the sweet peace of that time after my surgery had evaporated, and seemed now cruel illusion. I had been willing then to accept my losses because it was over and could have been worse. But it was not over, and now it was turning out to be worse than I had ever been warned it could be.

I suspected that what was interfering with my physical recovery was my emotional distress, my unfinished mourning and especially the unremitting burden of being always with Harl.

Indeed what sort of life was this? I had pinned too much on the move; now that it was done and there was nothing more to look forward to, reality was a fist in the stomach.

Though I felt physically worse than Harl did and was struggling to put in as much time as I could at the office for the support of both of us, he would not shop or do any household chores. The children were doing most of the shopping and housekeeping, and we were all eating a lot of tuna sandwiches and Campbell's soup. What I particularly wanted Harl to do during the days when he was home and I was not was unload and reload the dishwasher. He would unload but not reload it. Dizzy and exhausted, I repeatedly came home to a dirty kitchen. Sometimes I went so far as to cry about it. Harl was always solicitous about my tears and would try to comfort me as I lay weeping in my accustomed spot on the sofa, but the next day he still would not load the dishwasher.

Though my own finances were no longer secure, and I expressed to him that I was very frightened about this, he never willingly paid for anything. In restaurants he always looked pathetically at me, pushing a check across the table to me, indicating he did not have enough money.

His posture had begun to slump. Once complimented at the hospital for sitting straight as an arrow even when first propped up on the side of the bed, he now humped over with shoulders huddled together like some creature of no worth at all. Sometimes I would say with a razor edge of desperation, "Stand up; you're Harl Young!" and he would obediently straighten up. But once when I said that as he got into the car, I looked over at him a moment later and saw tears in his eyes.

That eroding of his self-esteem was the one thing I had most wanted not to happen. Was I in part responsible? I must be; I was nearly his only contact. His impressions of himself were coming through me.

Mostly I was still patient with him. But as spring rolled into summer and I was no better a scream formed inside of me, a deep ever-present unscreamed scream at his eternal silence. And there was murder in me too, because he sat there like a lump and did not talk to me. I wanted to scream *say something*, wanted to seize him and shake the words out of him, reach down his throat and rip them out. Sometimes I did give in enough to say, gently but with some irritation, "Harl, can't you say *anything?*" and he would stare back at me in mute misery, shrugging no.

* * *

Harl had two old bicycles that we had never been able to use while living in the mountains. He now began expressing that he wanted to get them repaired for riding. Watching bicyclists go by as we sat in the park, he would raise his hands over his head and clap, his gesture for joy that bound me to him as nothing else could do.

I did not think Harl could ride a bicycle. His right leg was much too slow. I gave the bicycles to a repairman as he requested, but I did not even think to tell him when they came back.

He spotted them one afternoon through the garage window as we sat on our back porch, and clapped his hands and wanted to try one out right then in the alley behind our house. I had just come home and just settled down to rest; I was dizzy and did not want to do this, and on top of that I had a sense of impending tragedy because I did not believe he could do it.

Balancing the bike as I had done when my children were learning to ride, I helped him try. But he was heavier than my children; on our third try the bike fell over on me and cut my leg.

Harl sat on the porch and wept. Because he could not ride the bike, or because I had gotten hurt? I had seen the tragedy coming; why had I not been able to keep it from happening?

Pressing a bandage to my leg, I thought suddenly that his

impression that he could ride a bike must have come from pedaling the stationary bike in physical therapy. Concrete thinking kept him from seeing the difference between this and actually balancing on a two-wheeler. How much it must have meant to him, watching the speed and freedom of those bicyclists in the park and imagining he could have that too!

Such a coper I was in practical ways, while inside feeling still like the aftermath of an earthquake....By the end of the next day I had located a three-wheeled adult bicycle for disabled persons, and ordered it from a Sears catalog.

Wanting the pain of the bicycle failure wiped out as quickly as possible, but also wanting to surprise him, I was too excited to keep it entirely to myself. I told Harl he had a present coming and that he was going to like it very much. His face lit with interest.

Cathryn and I unloaded the bike from the car and set it on the sidewalk, blue and shiny. I went to get Harl: "Come out, your present is here."

He went out and straight down the steps, his eyes locking on it. Something in his manner took me abruptly back in time to Cathryn's third birthday, when she as a tousle-headed barefoot waif had headed down some steps in exactly that same way to a shiny blue tricycle on the sidewalk. It was the same transfixed and greedy look, the same forgetting of the people around who had made the gift, the same total attention to action and object: go to the bike, ride the bike.

At three it was wonderful and appropriate; at fifty-five it was disquieting. He did not think to say thank you. My thanks would be his radiance when he was able to ride the bike. That was what I had wanted; I pushed away my vague disappointment. And I pushed away the thought that I had made him this three hundred dollar gift at a time when I was angry with him about money.

There was an occasional odd accuracy to Harl's speech. While I politely called the three-wheeler a bicycle, Harl always called it more accurately his *tricycle*.

Journal Entry, August 10

Harl was always an appreciator of beauty. But I see his appreciation going now to new depths, beyond what I can share. He can sit for hours in our tiny back yard, looking, pointing out with joy a bird's nest or "one perfect rose." He tries to show me cloud formations of unusual beauty, uses his hands to describe his delight with the shape of branches meeting between trees. One morning the skylight in our bedroom reflected one tiny leaf, and he noticed it and watched with indescribable pleasure as gradually a whole cluster of leaves began to be reflected. He spends hours alone at the park sitting in his car, looking.

Scientific to the end, he would not, will not even consider some of what I think of: life beyond life, reincarnation even, spiritual growth from one existence to another. To him the stroke has ended life.

He could be wrong. Even Albert Einstein is said to have been deeply religious. Beauty may be solace for its own sake, one of Harl's few remaining pleasures. But I think: could this thing have happened so that this wonderful, stubborn man might be brought to God through beauty?

I could not stand my illness. Nights I stared into the dark, dizzy even then without moving an inch, and wondered what in the world I could do. There was still so much impulse to care for Harl, but it broke like glass on my own illness. Given one wish, I would make myself well. Given two, I would make myself well and give Harl back his speech.

I wanted Harl but not all the time. How then to work out a more part-time arrangement? Harl's family members had surely been fortunate to have me in the picture. Could it be as simple as telling them I *would* not have him fifty-two weeks a year any longer? That if they loved him, they would have to start doing their share?

But his parents were eighty years old and could not care for him. Jeane was going through a divorce and was no longer financially secure, and it was she who primarily cared for their parents. Donna was not in good health herself, had a daughter in college and was looking forward to her husband's retirement in a few years. It was doubtful that she would want Harl living with them. And Harl was (or used to be?) different from his other family members, more sophisticated, wanting to travel and go to dinners and plays and otherwise have the kind of life only I could offer him.

Or could have offered him until now. Now I was dizzy all the time. Beaten down to my few feet of space on the sofa, I could not offer anybody anything.

His children would be the obvious solution, the ones who should be taking him for visits and if necessary helping to support him. But Harl had always said that although he loved his children very much, they were not his kind of people. I knew for sure he did not want to stay with them.

Realistically, *could* I make this a more part-time arrangement without putting him in a partial care facility? I cringed from the thought. He could not talk to the other residents; it would kill him.

Robin telephoned me several times a week. She pressed

me to get a break from Harl, to insist that he spend some time with his family. Encouraged by her, I called and told his sisters I wanted a month's vacation in October so Robin and I could take a trip together.

Robin and I planned to drive through the midwest, revisiting homes of our early childhood.

* * *

Strokes would be easier by far to cope with if the personality changes were more consistent, if one could say, "This person has the emotional nature of a five-year-old," and act accordingly. But what is most baffling is what flashes through when one least expects it, a part of him that is still a deeply feeling, deeply suffering adult human being.

Harl retained his gift for reading people, an intuitive quality that had always been a significant part of his personality. He also retained an adult sense of humor. This would seem almost certainly to depend upon abstraction, but it did not. He could appreciate a television comedian as much as ever, and could laugh even at jokes that entailed sophisticated word plays. I could only surmise that humor must have more to do with one's emotional sense of people than with abstract thinking.

Most confusing were the feelings he retained for me. I was trying to grasp that he had, as Kathleen warned me, lost the ability to put me ahead of himself. I also felt what she called loss of emotional depth in him, felt in a word that he loved me less. Yet I was repeatedly startled by how much he did at times seem to love me, how instantly responsive he could be to my feelings. Or was this just emotional lability?

Harl cried so frequently that I had to think either he was feeling very deeply or very superficially. Most confusing was that sometimes it seemed to be one and sometimes the other.

He had no interest in the newspapers except for the sports pages. But he cried every day over the sports pages. He cried before televised football games at the playing of "The Star Spangled Banner." Sporting events seemed to hold some special significance for him, perhaps reminding him of his own years of competing and winning. So was I to interpret this as deep grief over his losses, or as passing lability?

He cried over soap operas. But he also cried over deeper dramas, at appropriately moving lines where the audience is supposed to cry. Even back in that first year he had cried over the final volume of *The Life and Work of Sigmund Freud*, explaining to me that this was because of Freud's terrible final illness. Did his crying then indicate childish identification of the subject matter with himself, or a larger identification of himself with suffering humanity? Was he a child or an adult?

The trouble was he was both, or perhaps more accurately neither. I could not treat him as either and be entirely right. I could not wear myself out giving him constant consolation for what was often mere superficiality, but neither could I assume he was incapable of deep grief.

Sometimes in the nights I rolled over and held him, but that was more to comfort myself than him. Since the stroke he had rarely shown any desire for physical contact and never hugged me back. I could not tell that my holding him made any difference to him at all.

* * *

We had bought season tickets to the Central City Opera. I got on the phone and found people to go with us, old professional acquaintances of Harl's. We drove up the first Saturday of the season, Harl and I in the back seat where he sat in silence and I could keep my eyes closed to ward off dizziness. How enjoyable could this be for our friends?

The play was *A Desert Song*, that silly spoof of a romance with its achingly romantic music: *Oh, give me that night divine*....Harl and I were both weeping at the end. I wanted, wanted, *wanted*. Would it always be my most bitter regret that I let sex and romance slip away while I still had the youth and beauty to find them?

For him it was all over, and so he wept.

* * *

It had to happen eventually.

I knew him as the ex-husband of a friend, a man who was now dating another of my friends. Harl and I had a rare invitation to a party where he was present; I had gone outside for a little while to escape from Harl. Going back up to the party, this man and I entered an elevator together.

In the elevator he pulled me to him and kissed me. There was a moment of conscience as I thought of my two friends, then a heat that wiped out everything. In a back bedroom off the party, it was I who pushed it, reckless of interruption. He made love to me quickly and violently, too quickly but violently enough to set off two and a half years of pent-up longings. My hunger for lovemaking was so great that I wanted even pain; I muffled my cries against his chest and begged him to hurt me.

That night I dreamed I heard a beautiful strain of music in my deaf ear.

* * *

I had no illusions about my new lover. I hoped only for a sexual relationship and was surprised at what a pleasure it was to talk to him. I was as starved for male companionship as for sexual excitement, but for some reason I had hidden that need even from myself by disguising it as something sexual only.

Even more compelling was that he was physically affectionate, holding and touching me for hours even when we were not making love. My need for that seemed insatiable; I wondered how I had ever lived without it for so long. That was a deprivation that was not necessary, and I was angry at Harl for it.

So far I had not told Harl. Our agreement was that we were free to sleep with other people provided we did not lie to each other about it. I did not want to lie to him now. But I wondered if the fact of the stroke should not cancel out that agreement. He could no longer seek outside relationships of his own. He was frightened of losing me. If told, his mind might stick on it, so that he became unable to think of anything else. I could not judge how hurt he might be. Usually I thought so-called "protective" lies protected the liar more than the lied-to, but in this case I wondered if lying might not really be more kind.

For the time I managed to pull it off without telling him but without specifically lying either.

This man of course did not treat me well. I had not

expected him to. When he went weeks without calling, I felt briefly rejected but quickly moved on to someone else.

* * *

Harl's flight for his month-long visit with Donna and Jeane was held up for six hours, and finally cancelled.

The airport made me so dizzy that I could not see. Finally told we must wait another two hours for the rescheduled flight, I got us a table in a packed coffee shop, and some drinks and machine vended sandwiches. I had been crying off and on for hours; now I suddenly could not stop.

This separation that I had wanted seemed much harder on me than on Harl. All day there had been an odd vacancy about him, for me the worst part of this whole dreadful day. His eyes were devoid of life, empty of the light I loved, empty even of suffering. He had made no effort at all to talk to me.

Now I dripped tears onto my ham and cheese sandwich and pleaded with him to say something. His eyes drifted to me as he said absently, "Don't twy." But no expression returned to them.

I continued to cry.

* * *

Robin's Subaru had headrests positioned perfectly for me. I could spend most of the day with my head supported, almost eliminating my dizziness. I could enjoy the trip.

Spookily, at each house of our childhood we arrived just

as a current owner was coming into the driveway or walking around the yard. Robin had brought her baby book and showed them pictures of the house from the time we lived there. Everyone let us in.

The house in Pennsylvania where I was four. Playing in the sandbox (no longer there, but I could place where it had been), my mother coming onto the porch to call me in.

The house in Tennessee where I was five. The kitchen where I learned to skate (could it really have been so small?), rolling from table to counter and back, my mother cooking something and encouraging me.

The house in Indiana, the last place she lived. Then the cemetery, the grave so grown over we could not even find the flower container and had to get help to pry it open. Finally the flowers, yellow daisies accented by five large red daisies, one for each of her five children. Later, behind closed eyes, I would work out every detail, the gravestone itself, the inscription -

Marjorie Ruth
1911-1954

and the flowers behind it, triumphant.

It was easy to feel that she was there, happy that we had done this. Was it possible there might be a design in things after all, that Harl's wrecked life was only a passing shadow, that he would know speech and joy again? Conjuring up the flowers on my mother's grave, I could momentarily believe such things.

* * *

I had had Harl's car auto-transported to Austin so he could use it while he was there and drive himself home. He had been very taken with the adventure of that, his first independent travel since his stroke. His route was carefully marked out on a map, and he was armed with notes to cover every possible emergency. We had agreed that he would have me called each evening when he checked into a motel.

The first call came from a Howard Johnson's in Norman, Oklahoma. Harl was there and came on the phone. I asked him in some surprise how he happened to be in Norman, this not being a typical route from Austin to Denver. He started to cry, and I could not understand what he said.

The second call was from Roswell, New Mexico. Baffled by his circuitous route, I studied a map and concluded he must be losing his way. Later he would tell me he was missing the exits, which made sense considering his difficulty in switching his attention from one thing to another. But he was showing a good ability to adapt, getting closer to home each day even though by a peculiar route.

The third day I stayed home and waited for him, wild to see him. He arrived brimming with happiness, jaunty almost in the white canvas cap he had always worn for driving. His eyes glinted with triumph.

I lay beside him and held him for a very long time.

* * *

We sat together in the office of my company's lawyer, trying to get our finances untangled. In the clear-headedness of separation, I had reconsidered the reasonableness of our continuing fifty-fifty split of household expenses. This had been our arrangement on the Evergreen house, which we were now renting while hoping for an improvement in the real estate market. But since contributing his half of the down payment for the new house, Harl had had no money. Theoretically he was to pay half the monthly house payment, but since he had no money I was in practice carrying most of his share for him, while still letting him hold a half interest in the house.

Nor did it seem that tying all his money up in a house on which he would probably never collect the appreciation was a sensible thing for Harl to be doing at this point in his life. He no longer needed investments; he needed his money to spend. Our present arrangement was not working well for either of us.

Harl would not have had savings left to put into the house except that I had been largely supporting him ever since the stroke, to the tune of something over twenty thousand dollars, by continuing his salary from my company. So by paying him back what he had put down on the house, I would be effectively repaying money I had already given him.

But that was what I offered to do. I also offered to reduce his share of the house payment from one-half to one-third and to take over payment of all the utilities.

In exchange I wanted to terminate a buy/sell agreement for my company's stock. We had entered into this agreement before Harl's stroke. He had contributed five thousand dollars to the company's capitalization, thus owning approximately a one-third share. Our buy/sell agreement provided for each of us to buy the other's stock in the event of death and also for the company to buy out Harl's stock at an appreciated value on his sixtieth birthday.

Having continued Harl's salary for more than two years since he became disabled, I did not think it reasonable that I should also have to buy out his stock. Twenty thousand dollars in exchange for five was surely the best investment he had ever made. Harl had seemed to agree, and so here we were.

But now he was changing his mind. He had already taken my check for half his down payment on the house, and I had signed a promissory note for the other half, payable in one year. But all at once Harl would not sign the termination of the buy/sell agreement. He pointed to the paragraph to which he objected: he did not mind terminating the death buyout, which was as much to his advantage as mine, but he wanted to retain the buyout of his own stock at age sixty.

Could this be happening?

Of course it could; it was exactly the sort of thing Kathleen had been warning me about. But I had applied her warnings to smaller things--no window seats on airplanes, no help with cooking or cleaning. I had not thought about what a vulnerable position I put myself in by giving money so freely to someone who felt no need to be fair.

Upset enough to make an uncharacteristic scene right in the lawyer's office, I first shouted and then walked out. Even then I felt anxiety for poor Harl left embarrassed and unable to talk with the dumbfounded lawyer, but I was angry enough not to relent and go back.

I was not angry enough to leave him without a ride home. Someone would call him a cab; he would make it home, and my point would be made. But I could not do it. I waited by the elevators downstairs; outside the glass doors was my car. I had only to walk out and drive it off. But I would not do it. There were limits on free will; I was not free to abandon Harl. I was as dependent on this relationship as he was.

Elevators opened and closed. I waited by them knowing he would come eventually.

He came by himself, not at all surprised to see me, limping purposefully to the car as soon as he got off. He had known I would not leave him. More maddening even than the rest of it was his knowing that.

The money was important; the buyout would come due when I had all three of my children in college at once. But it was much more the emotional part that had me this upset. I did not leave the house for two days. I cried and pointed out the numbers to Harl and called him a double-crosser and said my heart was broken and I wanted to separate. He ignored me. He could not stand conflict and did not argue with me. He wanted only for me to be sweet again, to make his life comfortable again. But he was not about to give up that stock buyout.

On the third day he came to me suddenly smiling, holding theatre tickets in his hand. Tonight was one of our theatre nights; he was wanting us to be happy about it.

This theatre business had been a nightmare for me ever since my surgery. I could not enjoy it and never wanted to go. I occasionally suggested that I might not be well enough to go. On those days Harl would watch me hopefully all day, wanting so badly for me to go that he thought of nothing else. I knew I was an adult who was free to say no, but just once I wanted *him* to say, "You're too sick; let's not go." He never did, and I always went.

This time was no different. The plays were the highlight of his month; I went.

I had to keep my eyes closed through most of the play because the theatre made me so dizzy. Harl looked at me with concern and frequently patted my hand. Yet as we settled into the car afterward, he turned to me and asked brightly, "Wear are we doing do eat?"

I dropped my head onto the steering wheel and cried out,

not in anger this time but despair. "You *can't* think we're going out to eat. You *know* how bad I'm feeling."

He sat back abashed and said nothing else until after we were home.

But as we went to bed he succeeded in bringing it up, touching me to be sure he had my attention, his lips quivering with the effort of shaping his words. Normally he could not initiate any subject and only followed my conversational leads; he must have been thinking very hard about this.

What he said was something to the effect that we always went to dinner after a play. His face was taut, jaw knotted with the anxiety of wanting to get this across to me. Anger fizzled out in me like a balloon deflating.

He was right of course; what he said really was the problem. His mind got so stuck in patterns that he did not see reasons for breaking them. And that he had made this effort to explain himself proved he was not completely oblivious to my feelings; he seemed worse about that than he was because he could not talk about them.

Also: in the stock buyout business was there something perhaps deeper and better than selfishness going on in him, as with the wallet he guarded in his top drawer, some protection of his own basic security? To claim that security in this way, not backing down or passively going along--although in this instance technically wrong, could the root of that be something actually healthy?

I was lapsing in spite of myself, feeling a familiar slide away from what I had just been telling myself was Reality. So little was ever what it seemed; maybe reality was not really that bad. There was still Harl's gentleness, his occasional odd happiness, his simplicity. And that rapt attention he gave me, the expressiveness of his face, the light in his eyes. Even his terrible speech, reverberating in my brain as I fell asleep at night. Maybe all this was Reality too. Maybe it was enough to ask of living that I loved him.

* * *

An early December medical checkup confirmed what I suspected, that I still showed no balance compensation. For the first time Dr. M-- now admitted to me that I might never fully compensate, meaning I could remain dizzy permanently.

I found no words to say.

Home, I cried in a different way than I had cried in the nights after being first told I must lose my ear. Then I had sobbed until I could not breathe in the grief of irrevocable loss, but it had been a grief I knew would end, its very force a promise that in a short time I would dry my eyes and go on. Now I wept slowly, hopelessly, not in healing grief but in fear and horror.

Whether Harl "really cared" or not was not what mattered. What mattered was that he could not help me, and I had to help myself.

He came to bed from his evening of television, smiling as he climbed in beside me, looking inquiringly at me to see if I would say something. I had cried myself out; now I turned my head on the pillows that propped it, touched his hand and said it.

"I need you to go away for a while, Harl. To give me time to get well. I want you to spend three months with your family."

His smile vanished, replaced by a look of such dismay that at once a part of me wanted only to make it right for him, to take back what I had said. It was going to take every scrap of strength I had to go through with this.

"Harl, I love you. But I'm too sick to be taking care of you. I need to take care of myself. I need you to go away for a while."

As if relieved, he smiled happily again and gestured toward himself and around the room, taking in closet and bureau and bath. He was saying that I did not have to take care of him, that he would take care of himself.

I kept on. "Harl, you can't. I think about you all the time, I feel bad for you all the time--I need you to go away so I can try to get well."

He gestured again between himself and me, his face stricken with alarm and noncomprehension, saying words I could not understand but which I nevertheless understood. He was wanting to know how *he* stopped me from getting well.

What could I say? He was so concrete, he could not imagine a connection between my dizziness and what he perceived as his problems--the slowed hand, the weak leg, and of course the speech, which he indicated by gesturing with a grimace toward his mouth. What could *his* hand and leg and mouth have to do with my being ill?

I changed my tack a little; he had been a psychologist after all. "It's having to *cope* with it, Harl. I can't cope with being sick and cope with you too. You have to give me a break; you have to go for a little while."

My own increasing forcefulness seemed to trigger something similar in him. He abruptly said, "No!" and sat back looking suddenly sure of himself.

I had been so concerned about hurting him that this possibility had not occurred to me. Always I had thought I had a choice, that if I chose for him to go, he would go.

But now he seemed to have an inspiration. He hoisted himself out of bed and limped to his bureau, coming back with his address book in his hand. As I looked on in horrified disbelief, he began cheerfully looking through it for friends or former students with whom he could go and live.

He could deal with this only as something concrete, a *place to live*.

No wonder he did not appreciate me; he had no notion of what I did for him. He was coming up with people who had not visited him in two years, smiling eagerly at me as he pointed to their names. He had no comprehension that he required care, or any recognition that these were people who had abandoned him.

I sat beside him on the bed and thought there must be a limit to the sadness one human being could bear. His childlike innocence as always set off my protective feelings for him, and indeed under that fevered pitiful attempt to cope wasn't there surely terrible anxiety? I was pulling all his security out from under him. How terrifying would it be to know he could not talk and have to imagine himself alone in the world without a place to live?

But my own head spun miserably as always, and I knew I had to have this break.

Gently I pointed out the practical difficulties each person would have in putting him up. Tom had only a one bedroom apartment, Carla was just married and newlyweds never wanted company, Roberto lived up a narrow flight of stairs....After a while I said let's sleep and talk about it tomorrow, and I held him in the night although he would not then or ever hug me back.

The next day I called Kathleen, obtained the name of a partial care facility and arranged to visit it. If Harl would not go to his family, at least I could refuse to have him full time with me.

But that unspeakably terrible alternative proved

unnecessary, because that same day Harl came home from therapy, sat down with his cane across the arms of his chair and said quietly that he would like to spend his three-month "vacation" with Donna in Alabama.

He had come to his own sense of reality.

* * *

December moved inexorably as doom, Harl at the television, I dizzy on the sofa, the children muted and sorrowing for me. Donna had consented to Harl's spending the next three months with her. I would leave him with her in Austin at Christmas, to take to Alabama.

I had no confidence that I would become well in those three months or that I would ever feel capable of caring for Harl again. I had failed; this separation that threw its shadow on us was a proof of failure.

It was in the middle of that dreadful December that Harl came to me one day and said, the words carefully thought out and enunciated, "I don't *d'yub* d'yike I did." His eyes were full of fathomless distress; he was asking me for help.

I was not prepared. Obstacle crazed as much of my own life had been, nothing in it until now could have prepared me for the horror it would be to lose one's ability to love, and to know it. For a man like Harl who had loved more than most, for whom love included students and patients and treasured colleagues as well as the tender passionate physical love he had had for me--

I thought for the first time that suicide might really be appropriate.

Out of horror, I handled it badly. He had come to me to

talk about this. I should have acknowledged his feelings and talked about them with him; instead I denied them. I reminded him how he cried over a birthday card from Donna a few days before.

Doggedly lucid, he said that was because the card reminded him "of all the times before." And he began to weep.

After all my concern for his emotional coping, how could I deal with this so badly? It was the most important thing he had said to me since his stroke, the very crux of his life situation, and I continued to pretend ignorance. I said, "But you still love me, don't you?" A cruel question; how could he say no? He looked at me and I saw effort vanish from his eyes; he was giving up. He nodded, and returned to the television.

* * *

Robin was calling me almost every night. Alarmed by my mounting despair, she fed me lines to use on Harl and his family:

"You don't have to explain anything. Just say you *don't want to do it*. That is all you have to say."

Harl was wanting us to make our trip to Austin by car, stopping for a couple of days in Santa Fe. Robin exploded:

"You wouldn't enjoy one minute of that. You don't even want to go to Austin. Tell Harl you're putting him on a plane tomorrow, and you'll see him at Christmas."

I returned to the living room where Harl was watching television. I said, "I want you to take a plane to Austin tomorrow, and I'll see you at Christmas."

He said, "No."

We compromised by arranging to fly to Austin together on Christmas Eve.

On bright days I walked in the park, cold shocking my lungs. Too dizzy to see clearly and unable to walk a straight line, I feared falling on the ice. But there was a glint of sunshine on the snow, and out of despair the will to happiness pushed up in me.

I walked, and fought my own recurring hateful wish for Harl to die. I did not want to have this wish. Over and over I told myself it was not really my wish; I would not keep having it if only I could get some relief, see a break, see an end.

His silence was driving me mad. His tears, his passivity were driving me mad. In all these months that I had been ill he had not done one thing for me, not made me a sandwich, not offered to shop, nothing. He sat and looked at me by the hour, and even as something in me said *I love him*, I began to hate him. I was worn out with caring, sick to death of his crying over the sports pages, sick to death of him and all his suffering.

Sick especially of my own inability to hurt him. For that of course was the real trap. I kicked at snow drifts in frustration, my boots leaving futile jagged marks. We were not even married, I could walk out any time, but my own nature trapped me beyond how any outside circumstance could ever trap me. Where did it come from, this grit in me that recoiled in horror from the very thought of leaving him when he needed me?

And I loved him loved him loved him. Did I love him this much before the stroke? I couldn't remember. The scent of him, the feel of him, that certain light in his eyes; I was crazy with love for him. Robin said he was killing me. I thought I was dying of loving him.

So I wished for him to die, because I saw no other way out of this hopeless love that was killing me.

* * *

The children's intended Christmas visit with their father had for some reason fallen through. This meant that in going to Austin with Harl I would be leaving them alone on Christmas Day itself. The last thing I wanted to do was leave my children on Christmas Day, but with the three-month separation I had demanded from Harl about to begin, I could not bring myself to renege on taking him to Austin.

I did succeed in scheduling myself an earlier flight back on the 26th. This meant I would not see either of Harl's sisters. It was Jeane's first Christmas without her husband; she was coping herself by taking her children skiing. She and Donna would both be arriving late on the 26th.

So we were to spend Christmas in Jeane's house with Harl's eighty-year-old parents. They were crushed by Jeane's divorce and in grief over Harl's stroke (could I even imagine seeing such a thing happen to one of my children?), and I was much too ill to be the one who brightened things up. Harl was weepy as always, even more than usual.

Eternally, maddeningly dizzy, I lay on the sofa and reflected on this dark and silent house, this Christmas. I had tried to fill the silence by putting carols on the record player. They seemed a mockery, shocking in this scene of hopeless loss.

Journal Entry, Christmas Day

It is no use; we hear no angel voices. Such a sadness I have never known. Harl's parents old and heartbroken. Jeane's house shattered and empty. Me leaving Harl, the best thing I ever had.

After two and a half years and the destruction of my own health, what have I really been able to do for him? His grief is as deep as ever, mine more so. I see us all aging in loneliness, dying miserable and grisly deaths. What will mine be? Cancer probably, like my mother. Will I have anyone to support me as I have tried to support Harl?

Children growing up and leaving. **All of the children ran from your arms.** *Even Cathryn going away to college in a year and a half. What will become of me then?*

"Silent Night" on the record player. Memories of early childhood when Christmas was so beautiful and full of warmth and hope. I have not been able to keep it so.

Someone said **nostalgia is a swindler's trick.** *But also* **there is a time for love and a time for remembering.** *How does remembering differ from nostalgia? Can you learn to remember without pain?*

Harl so sad. Just brought out the video of his grandchildren, his Christmas present from Cindy. Wanting us all to watch it, still trying to create some happiness. I couldn't get the VCR to work, finally told him Jeane would make it work when she gets back. Enough hope to live on till tomorrow? He pretended it was all right.

How much that video must mean to him, that he would

think to bring it. Grandchildren with whom he will never talk, who will never know him.
  Amado Pena poster on Jeane's wall:

> *with that from the*
> *earth, beauty I will*
> *create. with that*
> *beauty, my soul I*
> *will give....*

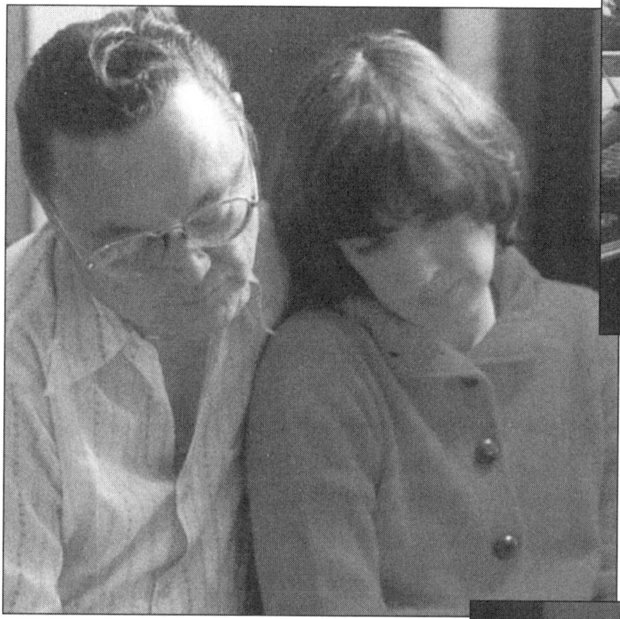

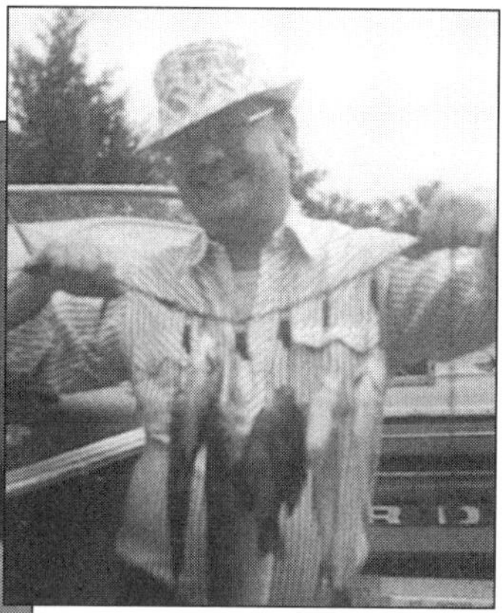

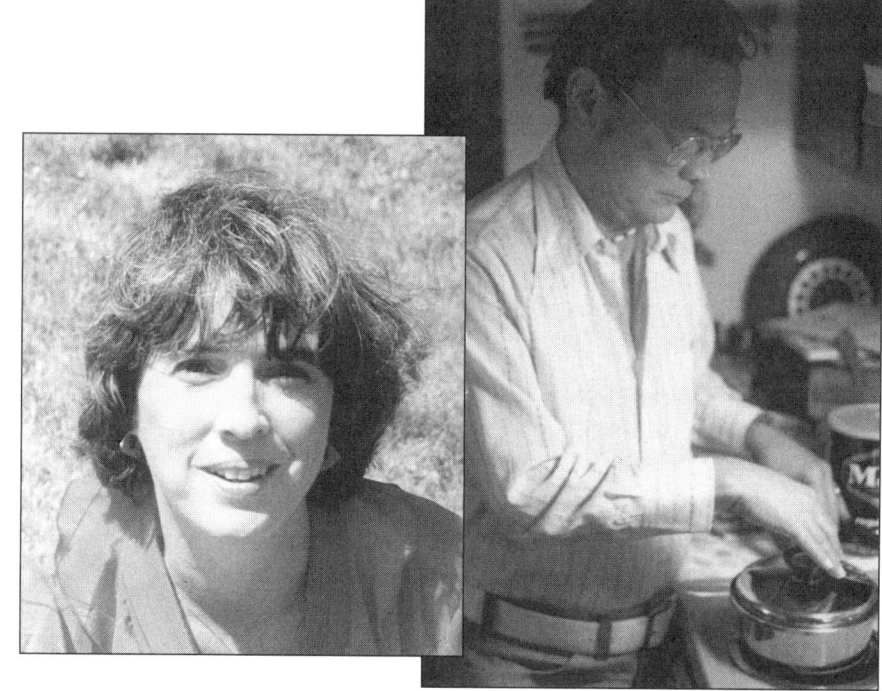

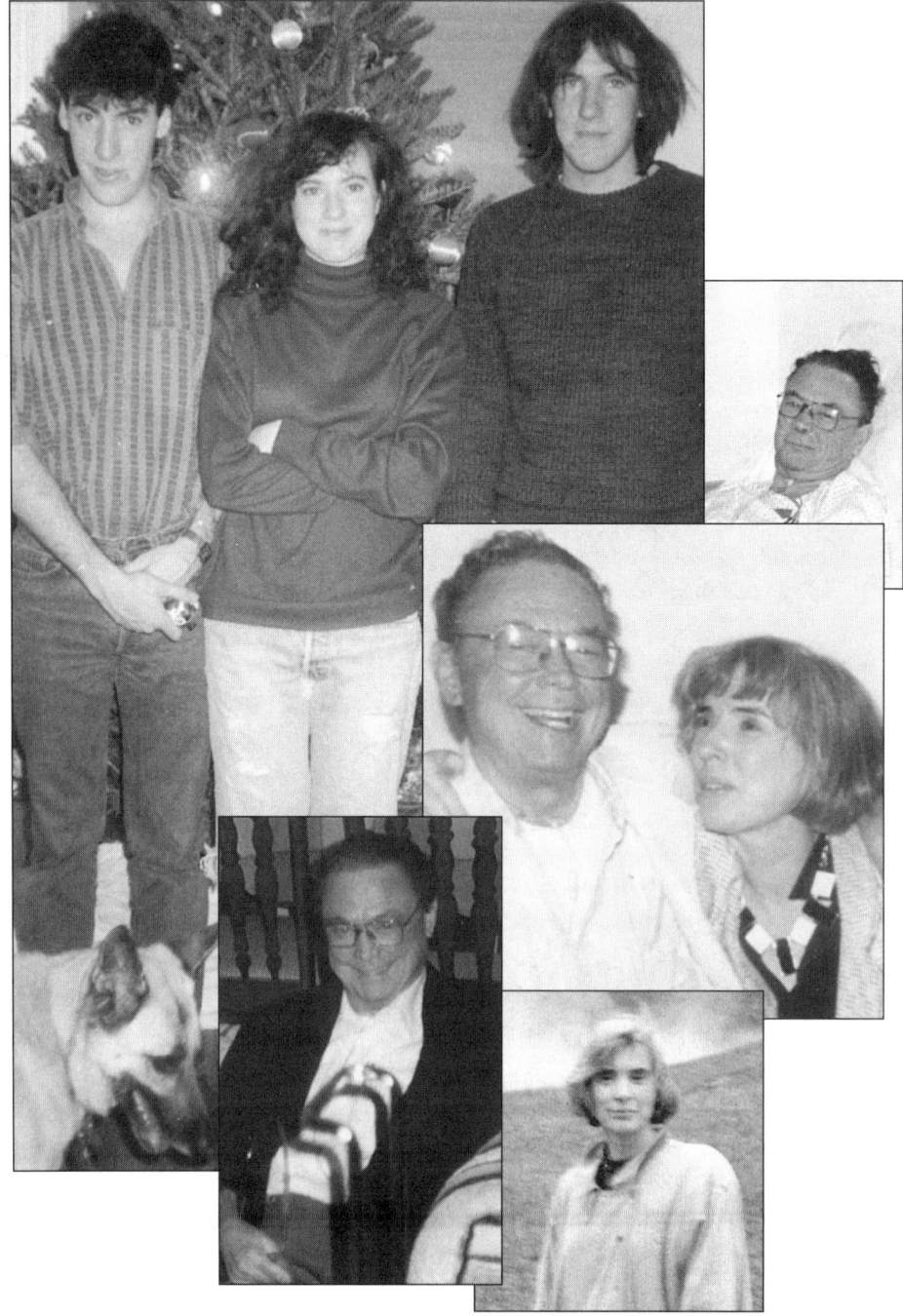

CHAPTER EIGHT

Loneliness is a condition of human life, an experience of being human which enables the individual to sustain, extend, and deepen his humanity.

---Clark Mousakas

To be alone is unendurable.

---Judith Viorst

  Home, I did not feel better. What had become of the oh-so-competent woman of the hospital visits, of the early months in Evergreen, arranger of therapists and attendants and evenings out, buyer of cars and bicycles? She huddled now shivering under piles of blankets, half deaf and always dizzy, too depressed to lift her head from the pillow for long enough to make herself breakfast.
  Had I forgotten his smile, his sitting warm beside me for coffee in the mornings, his rapt attention to my every word? Why had I sent him away?
  The stroke had been done to us, my tumor had been done to us, but this separation was nothing but my own appalling choice.
  Bring him back then? Call and he would be on the plane in a day, beaming as someone wheeled him down the ramp to meet me, ready as always to resume our life.
  I couldn't; I was too ill. Even to toss now on the pillow

thickened my head with wooze. I was so ill that if I did not improve I would never have anything like a normal life. And I had not improved at all that I could tell, in at least four months.

But had I been thinking this much about suicide before Harl left? I didn't think so. Now the idea of it was always idly on my mind, not a consideration exactly but like a daydream. How would I do it if I were going to do it? Running my car in the garage until I quietly passed out was the most painless and appealing method but made intent too obvious. For my children's sake, I would have to make it look like an accident. Driving my car off a mountain would involve too much fear and pain, an agonizing death. I could never do it.

Besides, Cathryn at least still needed me. I could not betray my closeness to Cathryn.

When my children were older and on their own, and if I was still dizzy, then perhaps I could use the garage method. Projected into the future, it seemed a more real possibility.

* * *

I was sleeping regularly with my current lover: driving over one or two evenings a week to his house where he met me at the door, eyes quizzical, arms already reaching. We fell on each other, we were in bed in five minutes.

There was no relationship developing, no sense that he was personally important. Just the grinding of belly on belly, and the moment when I would no longer know that I was dizzy and no longer care that Harl had had a stroke.

Might one go on living just for this?

* * *

During that dreadful December I had finally told Harl of my involvement with other men. It did not seem possible to keep it from him indefinitely, and I did not want whatever hurt he would feel to be compounded by being lied to. But a day later I found him lying with his arms wrapped around himself as if in complete grief. He would not turn over to look at me.

When I pressed him to talk, he said, "It dot doh pahlt and it dot my pahlt. But I dan't dand it anymow."

Compelled as always to try to cheer him up, I pointed out that much of the time he seemed fairly cheerful. He answered, "I ondy at dat way."

Certain that I had made a dreadful mistake, I talked about it with Bob--. He was not so sure.

"By telling him the truth, you've let him tell you the truth. He's telling you he's been faking. Maybe you need to know that."

Both of us faking? But what did that mean, and what would I do if I entirely believed it?

I remained unsure that truth was worth that much suffering. But as with other things, Harl seemed to adjust quickly. His letters from Mobile repeatedly asked questions about who I might be sleeping with but did so in a superficial, almost socially inappropriate way. I could not tell whether there was deep feeling there.

* * *

On a Sunday I called him. He was watching a football

game and seemed happy. Kathleen had predicted a certain out of sight, out of mind quality about him: "A five-year-old becomes very preoccupied with what he sees in front of him. Occasionally there may be the thought--`where's Mommy?'--but as long as his needs are being met, he will be content."

Was he, then? Content with Donna and his drink and his game, content without me? My eyes still turned to the chair where he had sat all those months staring at me. Its emptiness now brought on a sick feeling in my stomach, a choke of tears rising in my chest.

He could not talk on the phone long; he could manage only the most concrete conversation. He was happy; wasn't that what I had wanted? I said, "I miss you."

He said, "I mid doo too!"

I said, "Goodbye," and he said, "Dood bye-bye!"

And at the last moment he said, wistfulness coming mournfully over the wires, "I d'yub you!"

* * *

Kathleen had brought me to her house for coffee. We had just visited the partial care facility, to help me decide whether Harl's staying there was really a possibility. Now she brought me coffee in a silver service, pouring it into tiny flowered china cups. I went at it like a drug, the nearest thing at hand to make me feel a little better.

I simply could not do this thing. The place was as good as such places probably can be, not bad for an older couple or even for a single but sociable older man or woman wanting some security. There were small two-room apartments with balconies and views of the mountains; there was an attractive dining area with individual tables, and there was even a quite lovely atrium that had made me almost able for a moment to imagine Harl being there. Someone had taken the trouble to make that atrium beautiful; Harl had to have beauty.

But compared to living in our house with me, the place could only be a loss. Not just a small loss but a great devastating loss. I had tried to picture him in one of the chairs in the dining room, but saw only his look of hunger for my every word.

Kathleen talked of his making friends there, but how could he when he could not talk? I said almost dreamily now, because too much grief and horror threw me into dream states, "It would kill him."

Kathleen said, "You have not been able to recover your own health. That is evidence enough you cannot cope with this as it is."

Was it though? Kathleen and Bob-- and I were all quick to assume my baffling non-recovery was because of Harl, but actually I didn't have a scrap of evidence for that. Maybe I was putting both of us through all this agony for nothing.

Everyone was too much on my side.

I said tonelessly to Kathleen, "I would have to visit him several times a week. And have him stay with me on weekends."

Kathleen said, "Oh, I don't think you'd need to visit that much. Maybe at first, but in a little while he would settle in. Once a week would be plenty."

She was envisioning more of a break than I was, my making a life for myself without Harl. Would it finally come to that, the care facility really a dumping ground after all? A place for Harl to wait conveniently out of sight until he died?

I took a quick look ahead at that life without Harl that Kathleen had in mind for me. She imagined friends and new men and all the stimulation Harl held me from. To me it looked like a nuclear winter.

Astonishing how my mind kept providing me remembered lines of poetry to match whatever was going on. This time it was a phrase from a Shakespeare sonnet that I had not read since freshman English some twenty-five years before. *Bare ruined choirs where late the sweet birds sang.*

Kathleen said, "You had a relationship that was based on ideas and suggestions. Now you have nothing like that, and you have a person who is completely predictable. It is only natural for you to wonder how much longer you will have to do this, when it is going to end."

Only natural to be wondering when he would die.

I said I wished Harl had been more receptive to counseling with her. She said, "By the time I met him, Harl was already set in a pattern. That pattern included you being his caretaker and also his counselor. He was living there in the mountains, going to the office and to therapy and having you to meet his every need. There was nothing to motivate him to work with me."

I had not thought of it that way before, the setting of a pattern and how a stroke victim would settle into that. All those early months of so much dedication, all that bright love my memory still treasured, had been at least in part a terrible mistake. I had set Harl up to believe this would be his life forever, and now I was finding I could not keep it up.

But I had not known I would become ill. I had not even known I was setting a pattern, because I had not understood how changed he was and how prone to settling into patterns. Wearily, I wondered how such good intentions could possibly turn out to be so destructive.

I said I guessed I should have started Harl out in a partial care facility when he first left the hospital. He would have accepted it then and not been hurt. Now I had got myself in so deep that I was still not sure I could get myself out.

Kathleen said, "At the beginning he was not capable of it. *You* have brought him to the point of independent living. He would not be functioning anything like as normally as he is if he had not had you."

So my effort had not been entirely wasted after all.

She continued. "And I do not mean any criticism of you, but you have been extraordinarily good for Harl, much better than anything most stroke patients ever have. You have done everything possible to restore him as nearly as possible to his former life. And one consequence of that is that he has had very little motivation to do that for himself."

She was saying that now, if he was forced to, he might acquire that motivation. I downed a third cup of coffee, reaching for the pot to pour a fourth. I was after all considering only a part-time separation. I still meant to have him much of the time with me, most of the weekends and at least another night during the week. But not sitting there staring at me always every minute, with no escape ever.

I said *If only he could adjust and not be always pulling me into his grief, perhaps I could stand it.*

Kathleen said, "I just don't think a man like Harl ever adjusts."

* * *

Letters came, as baffling as Harl himself. Donna had told me how upset he was over the explosion of the Challenger, the sudden horrifying death of seven crew members as America watched on television. He cried for days; when a later news magazine came full of pictures and stories about it, Donna hid it.

I thought how relieved I was that I did not have to be the one to cope with that. Then his letter, written on that day:

27 Jan 86

~~Hi~~ Pretty Thing,
　I finished all the ~~💲~~ bills for this time! I just got there last night Oh -- the last words were "get the bomb, exploded" the space craft!
　I got the ~~birthday~~ birthday birthday present last night for you. Its' kinda purty, difficult for you.
　— I've caught him last

> night — I just can't get them out of my mind — that McGuge, or whatever her name was, getting it! Thousands of Turks sobbing their hearts out today — & whatever must go on in the minds of children — —

So much feeling. So like his old self to care so much, and on such a feeling level, about world events. But was this also his superficial lack of emotional control? We all felt sad, but he could not stop crying. And there was a typical mixture of the deep with the banal. Yet the remark about the children, something I had scarcely thought of, so sensitive and aware. Who was he, whom was I dealing with?

Whom was I about to betray?

January was slipping by; something was going to have to be done. I had told Harl I would come to Mobile in February to spend my birthday with him. That would be the time to talk to him about the care facility, but I felt no more capable of doing it now than I ever had.

My clothes hung on me like oversized hand-me-downs; since Harl left I had become unable to eat. Knowing that not eating would make me more dizzy, I struggled with myself every morning, pouring a bowl of cereal and sitting down to it with spoon determinedly in hand. Some days I could get down a few bites. Others revulsion would so overtake me that I threw the whole bowl down the garbage disposal and settled for a glass of milk and a vitamin.

I had always been so impressed by Harl's idealism; only since his stroke had I begun to realize how idealistic I was myself. No one could have approached this thing with greater propensity to take emotional distress and elevate it to a philosophical level. It was the *dailiness* of life with Harl that ground that effort out of me, that ground me down. I wanted to be a phoenix rising from the ashes, but I was jittery with losses and maddened by years of efforts that seemed never to work enough.

And I was ill, crazed by my own unabating dizziness. The garage would be the best way, yes. Say around two in the morning when I would be least likely to be apprehended. I would take blankets and a pillow and bourbon and ice. Maybe a book, though I might be thinking too seriously about myself to read. I would turn on the car engine and lie down on the back seat with my head propped up, so I could die as undizzy as possible. I should have a hose to speed it up and make interception less likely, but I did not know where to get one. Could one go into a hardware store and say, "I want a hose about six feet long and just a little wider than an auto exhaust pipe"?

Out of my struggle to reestablish relationships with people other than Harl, I regularly got dressed up enough to go to lunch with my friend Andrea. Sometimes being with other people made it more possible for me to eat; other times I still could not eat beyond the first few bites, but even that was better than I managed at home.

A psychologist herself, Andrea had been one of Harl's students and was being supervised by him when he had his stroke. She had never visited or done anything for him after the stroke, but she had been my most consistent friend. I struggled with that ambiguity, a part of me shutting down against her even as I appreciated her attention to me.

It was Andrea who suggested over a plate of Chinese food that I should look further into the possibility that I had some brainstem injury.

"You don't know what they might have *done* in there. Maybe they cut something they shouldn't have."

I was confused, blinking through my dizziness from across the table. "But they did such a good job, they didn't paralyze my face."

But Andrea was suddenly inspired. "*I* know what you should do. You should go get neuropsychological testing with Jim--."

Jim-- was someone with whom Andrea, recently and traumatically divorced, had had a brief disappointing romance. He was also the neuropsychologist to whom my company always referred clients with suspected brain injuries.

Was it just my dizziness that made my head so muddled? This was not the first time I had been confronted by my own occasional startling lack of judgment. Or by other subtle signs of brain dysfunction: my repeated forgetfulness of things that had just been said in company staff meetings, my peculiar inability to find my way around in stores or malls. When I routinely referred clients to Jim-- for evaluation of just those kinds of symptoms, how had I not thought to refer myself?

* * *

The park was empty except for me, wind blowing snow hard into my face as I pulled my scarf up tighter and trudged against it. Soon I would round a bend and get the wind behind me; then I could lift my head some and look around the park although I still had to watch my feet a lot to keep my balance.

Walking was no longer just for escape and pleasure but an outcome of my evaluation with Jim--, an exercise regime of activities known to stimulate cerebellum development in babies: crawling, rolling, walking, swinging.

The swinging I could do at the park playground. That part was fun except in cold and snow.

The walking was to be for an hour a day, concentrating on keeping an oppositional arm swing. One of my most glaring symptoms of cerebellum injury had been loss of a normal oppositional arm swing; without realizing it, I had been walking with the arms swinging together.

Other symptoms were enumerated in Jim--'s report: impaired concentration, loss of short-term memory, loss of spatial comprehension, a fine tremor of the left hand. And fatigue, and dizziness.

Especially dizziness. The injury was diagnosed as "mild," presumably from the necessary scraping of the brainstem during surgery, and mild enough that most of the symptoms might still spontaneously resolve. But even mild cerebellum injury could cause severe dizziness when combined with loss of an ear.

The wind was crosswise now; I could turn my head to the right and look across the frozen pond to trees bent with snow, beyond them a stretch of earth and sky that even now brought a longing lump to my throat. My life had turned to nightmare through little fault of my own, but it was still up to me to turn it back. Partial separation from Harl was what I wanted; I thought I could live with that. Weekdays at the partial care facility, weekends with me. Where I would still care for him, sleep with him, talk to him, listen to him.

Still have him warm in my bed, still see that light in his eyes when he looked at me.

Especially if these exercises worked and I could stop being dizzy, it was a compromise that might let me be happy again. The nightmare now was having to tell him.

I rounded another curve; the wind behind me, I could lift my head and look straight forward. It is not possible to keep obsessing on one subject every minute of a day; the mind must sometimes drop it and open up. In the momentary relief of that, I reached for some new thought big enough to keep the obsession out. But there was only my own loneliness and the piercing spiritual feeling in natural beauty, and all I could do with those was murmur a prayer to a God in whom I did not believe. *Help me.*

And as I trudged toward the next curve that would bring me back into the wind and on my way toward home, the words came unexpectedly to my lips that would be my whispered prayer through all the coming months of solitary walking: *Take this anger from me.*

* * *

In the midst of getting ready for my trip to Mobile, I had another idea. The rheumatic fever that damaged Harl's heart valve and eventually resulted in his stroke had occurred while he was in the Navy. Was it possible he could still qualify for V.A. disability benefits?

When I learned there was no time limit on application and that Harl almost certainly would qualify, I could scarcely believe I had not thought of this sooner. I got the application in before I left.

On the way to Mobile I was stopping in Richmond to spend some time with Robin.

I talked to Robin endlessly, repeating the same quandaries over and over--*he will be so hurt, I can't do it, I am so sick, I can't not do it*--and she was endlessly patient. She accompanied me in my exercises, walking beside me and helping me check my arm swing. At home the Washington Park playground was five minutes away; here there were no playground swings, so Robin instead bundled both of us in coats and rocked with me on her front porch swing. Our breath turned to steam in the biting cold; we wrapped scarves around our faces and swung and talked.

Robin interpreted my agony over hurting Harl as an immature belief that I must always please other people. She hammered home her conviction:

"If it bothers you this much to go to Mobile, don't go. Call him and tell him by phone. You don't have to go."

And, "If you are having a bad time there, call me and come right back. You don't have to go through this. You don't have to do anything you don't want to do."

Robin herself was of course the kindest person alive, the oldest sister of our traumatized family, very disinclined to hurt anyone. Witness her swinging here beside me, her lips blue with cold. Coming from her, these words had a depth I never felt in the *look out for number one* self-help books of the seventies.

But what this finally had to come down to was my own choice. I was going to do this unspeakable thing to Harl because that was my choice.

I got on the plane to Mobile feeling I must surely die on the way. No one could live an hour with this much anguish.

All to no point, because I didn't have to. Sometimes reality is better than appearance; sometimes when one says, "Maybe it isn't this bad," it isn't. Harl and I had already turned a corner. What was waiting for me in Mobile was the beginning of joy, and closeness, and the most precious caring love I could ever know.

CHAPTER NINE

Consider the courage in all that and behold the man.

---Vladamir Nabokov

My eyes were seeking him as I came off the plane, finding him at once, then riveting to him. There was the slightest mist of tears in his eyes; I saw the effort he was making not to cry. His face trembled with love and fear, his body so tensed with hope that it seemed that frail structure could not possibly hold so much.

Kathleen had been wrong; even Harl himself when he said out of his own numbing despair, "I don't love like I did," had been wrong. I moved to him to hold him; I could not look away even to say hello to Donna.

He had gained a little weight; my arms found his body a little rounder. But mostly what I felt was all that love and hope and fear pressing out of him. He hugged me back hard, his cheek warm against mine, the familiar scent of him bringing tears to my own eyes.

He had not been able to speak, because of his struggle not to cry. In the car as his arms circled me he said what he had been wanting to tell me, the words of hope as carefully rehearsed as they were poignantly inaccurate: "I hab a better *voice* now."

Crying, I said, "I can tell," and he said, "So dyet's doe

home and delebwate!" and we held each other all the way there.

Donna had been wonderful for Harl. The two of them had gone sightseeing, spent a week in Donna's condominium in Florida, even gone to Mardi Gras. With more chance to speak, his speech had improved.

But I was what he wanted. He sat by me on the sofa touching and looking at me the whole evening, held me and made love to me the whole night.

Mornings I had coffee with Donna before beginning my exercises. The exercises had not yet taken effect; my head was still heavy with wooze. Donna and I sat in our bathrobes at her kitchen table and talked about Harl and my inability to continue full-time care of him.

Because I still knew I could not. But telling him seemed more impossible than ever.

Donna could not help but see how ill I was, but she too was terrified about Harl's reaction. She told me the emotional state he was in the night before my arrival:

"Bonnie, I think he would *die* without you."

Harl got up every day in time to watch my crawling and rolling exercises. I had written him about them; bursting with excitement at this hope for me, he had shared that letter with Donna. It was becoming hard for me to believe that I had actually thought he did not care.

My hour of walking I did around a single block, fearing I would get lost if I went anywhere else. The oppositional arm swing was getting easier. I could hardly see, but I could see that Mobile was beautiful in February, fragrant and blooming with a moist springtime warmth in the air. If such beauty could exist in the world, surely happiness was possible?

The one obsessive thought was always with me, hammered into every step I took: *how* could I tell him?

Out of the thought of having to admit to Robin that after all my endless agonizing I had not said anything, I finally mustered the courage to do it. Just once, as we lay in bed on the next to last night of my visit, I said ever so tentatively that perhaps we should live apart some of the time after he came home, because I still did not feel physically able to care for him full time. He replied blissfully, "Then find me a place to live." And I briefly mentioned the care facility, stressing that I meant it to be only part-time, that we would still spend our weekends together.

He was so intuitive, he must have read me as well as I did him in that moment at the airport. He was not threatened; he knew I loved him. And in this time apart he too had been rethinking our life, and knew that what he wanted was to be with me.

*   *   *

I had two more months at home before Harl was to come back. Each morning I resolutely put on scarf and gloves and boots and set off for the park. My swing creaked back and forth over the dirty ice, the park as usual empty except for me. Snow stuck to my lashes; I swung and thought of Harl.

His letters were indicating astonishing equanimity with my suggestion of living apart, though he was thinking more of an apartment than a care facility. I was afraid of that. Since his stroke he had resolutely refused to cook or do much of anything else for himself. He had never shopped, and if I was too ill to cook, he would go to bed without eating.

With no one else to care for him, I could be more drained by keeping him in an apartment than home with me. Would I be always checking on him to make sure he was eating?

And I could not imagine him spending so much time absolutely alone. I did not like the location of the care facility, too many high traffic miles from my house. But there he would have meals provided, and the constant community of other people. There I would not have to be always worrying about him.

Since my visit to Mobile, my suicide fantasy had changed to joint suicide. We would go to the car together. We would take drinks and pillows and blankets and lie in the back seat, holding each other. That way I would not have to have him move out. It seemed a perfect solution; why had I not thought of it sooner?

His letters came:

11 Mar 86

Dear ~~Honey-Put~~,
Went to the ~~B~~ Perdido ~~Sea~~ area of ~~Gulf Shores~~! It must be crazy to think of you all the time we are seeing such sights I think of you all the time!

* * *

Harl went with Donna to visit Jeane in Austin and from there again drove himself home. I watched through the patio doors as he came up the walk, not yet aware of being seen, limping as fast as he could go. His expression was so nakedly full of hope that I had to open the doors and go to him. His cheek hollowed just where I remembered, his skin warm on my lips and sweet smelling as always.

We had finished our hours of holding each other on the bed; now he sat by me where I lay as usual with my head propped up on the sofa. Though better, I was still not out of the woods on my dizziness.

Harl had something he wanted to say to me, something he had obviously been thinking about and rehearsing for some time. He spoke with transparent anxiety, gesturing around him at the house to illustrate. What he said was something to the effect that I had been doing "all the work" and that this "didn't seem reasonable." There was genuine puzzlement on his face; he truly did not understand how or why that pattern had developed.   Donna too had done everything for him, so this was not a matter of his having had practice doing things for himself. It was something he had thought up and thought through all on his own.

He got out the words he had been rehearsing. "I want to *help* dyou," accompanied by a gesture of flexing his muscles, showing strength.

That post-stroke inability to hide his feelings lent a profound simplicity to everything he said. I loved him in that moment with as pure a love as I had ever known, and I also knew I had to separate from him.

We visited the care facility, and Harl did not like it at all. Its distant location was one problem, the old age of most of its residents another. He continued to speak instead of finding an apartment.   We discussed it on Sunday morning in my bed.

Trying to be concrete, I pointed out that the care facility provided meals. He had thought about that and said he wanted an apartment "near a cafeteria" so he could eat whenever he wanted. This was something he had thought of that I had not. The care facility served dinner only from four to six; Harl liked to eat late.

The thought of his eating in a cafeteria made my heart crunch. He would eat in a cafeteria even as I set a dinner on my table?

Still being concrete, I pointed out that he had not shopped or cooked since his stroke and that eating all his meals out would be very expensive. He considered that seriously and said he would cook. I pointed out the isolation of a single apartment as opposed to the community of the care facility. He expressed skepticism about the kinds of friends he could make there and about being so far from me. He gestured between us; especially he wanted to be close to me.

He also wanted something of the upper middle class lifestyle that suited him, a place near the park, a place of some elegance. There was still a personality in him, too much of one to make this an easy choice.

Later he sat next to me on a playground swing and pointed to a building across the park, his eyes turning inquiringly to me, the inflection of his voice showing a question. "I tould d'yib dere?"

That concrete thinking can become endearing. He had the innocence of a four-year-old and twisted my heart in the same way.

I said that building would probably cost too much, but we could look at it. He stared at it across the park and began to be excited; when I called the manager, he watched me with agonized suspense. The building was part of the Park Lane Condominiums, just six blocks from my house. The cost was higher than for the care facility but within his range if he got any V.A. disability, and I was sure he would get at least some.

He had to rely on me for cost decisions; he had no notion of what he had.

We went to look, and he grew more excited. It was a very secured building; a doorman could be reached by the pressing of a button and there was safe underground parking. One apartment was available on the twentieth floor, with a balcony and a spectacular view of the city. Harl limped about pointing and beaming, feverish with delight but still looking to me for my consent. He understood this choice involved me too; he would not make it without me.

How wonderful it would be to have him here, just six blocks from me. I capitulated; he took the apartment.

Harl did these things:

- Made his own list of furnishings he needed to buy.
- Went alone to Sears and bought a coffee pot, kitchen utensils, sheets and a comforter. Later bought a peach colored tablecloth to match a peach color in the comforter.
- Went to a garden center and bought a plant and hanging planter.
- Did his own grocery shopping.
- Did his own immaculate housekeeping.
- Cooked for himself.
- Cooked for me; lamb stew one night, glazed Italian sausage another, bacon and eggs for breakfast when I stayed over.
- Watched the newspaper for events he and I could attend: a movie series at the Performing Arts Center, a flower arranging class at Denver Free University, a Famous Author Lecture Series at the Lowenstein Theater.
- Met another stroke victim at physical therapy, learned he also lived in the Park Lane Condominiums and invited him

to watch a Sunday football game.

- Made love to me at least once a week.

Here in his apartment, with the meals he cooked for me, I began to be able to eat again.

* * *

His speech therapy must have been focusing on Fs and Vs. At my house for a Sunday morning in bed, I noticed the sudden new effort he was putting into Fs and Vs. He would stop in mid-sentence, repeating a word to get them right. And he did get them right. I had not previously seen this kind of carryover from his therapy. Until now I could never have deduced what sounds he was working on.

I sat by him with my head propped on pillows, to postpone getting dizzy. With my exercises, and also perhaps because I was eating again, I had just begun to wake up in the mornings undizzy. With movement dizziness returned; by the time I made coffee and got back to bed it was on me. But if I propped my head and sat *very* still, it would almost go away again.

We sipped our coffee and talked, Harl carefully enunciating those Fs and Vs. I had shown him an announcement of a department store warehouse sale. He read through it and showed me items he wanted, carefully circling them: a twenty-seven inch television, a VCR, a microwave.

I asked if he really wanted that large a television. And since he could still watch movies several times a week at my house, was he sure he wanted a VCR?

He answered happily, "Why not?" And circled a gas barbecue grill for his patio.

In a Spiegel catalog he had marked a gorgeous king-sized brass bed. We had always managed on a queen-sized bed for the two of us. Was he sure he wanted a king-sized bed?

All his old love of life was going into that apartment. He answered happily again, "Why not?"

The prices at the warehouse sale were too good to pass up. I had agreed to take him to it, though I had misgivings about what the place might do to me. Large and crowded places made me dizzy, especially when I had to look around for things to buy.

Harl clapped with happiness as we began to get dressed. He had marked about a dozen items in the catalog.

The sale was too dreadful to say. Mobbed, it was in a room so large that I went faint the moment we walked in. There was no way Harl could walk around a space this large; it would take him hours. A sales manager took pity on him and found him a bench, then took me to each of our marked items. He did not know I too was ill, but in consideration for Harl he rang up the sale himself so I would not have to stand in line.

In the car as we left the parking lot Harl touched my leg and unexpectedly said, "Dant dou, Donnie." And added very carefully, "I douldn't ab - *av* done it widout dou." There were tears in his eyes.

It was the first time since his stroke that he had thanked me.

*   *   *

The V.A. disability came through, an award that doubled his income and included $17,000 in back benefits.

He was in the hospital when I told him, one of many sudden hospitalizations for congestive heart failure. So far these episodes had always occurred when he was with me, and I was able to get him to a hospital in time. But they were so quick, starting with complaints of being cold which with his poor circulation were not at all unusual, then turning in an instant to teeth chattering chills that sent me flying to a phone for Dr. Friedman. I would get him to the hospital wrapped in a blanket, teeth clenched against the chattering, so blue in the hands and gray in the face that nurses would ask me in dismay, "How long has his color been that bad?"

I could not tell them. Was this my habitual obliviousness, not seeing these deteriorations until he hit the crisis stage? But his color was often bad, and he was always cold. I was desensitized from living with this for so long.

Today he was looking good again, color back in his face though his hands were a mass of bruises from the I.V.s. I had come early in barely contained excitement, bursting to tell him.

I stood at the foot of his bed. "You have some *good* news."

He looked at me alertly. I felt the smile spread across my face. "You've been awarded *total* disability by the V.A."

He took a long breath as it sank in, then screwed up his face and began to sob. I sat down on the bed and hugged him, whispering happily, "I *knew* you'd cry!"

Now he had some money, and all the deep generosity of his nature could flower again.

Because he had some money, he could browse through catalogs picking out small items to enrich his home: a green and brass desk lamp, a tablecloth in the peach color that ran through all the rooms and made him smile and clap his hands.

Because he had some money, he could reach like his old

self for a restaurant check, waving no at me as I made a move to pay my part, the contentment in his smile saying he wanted to do this for me.

Because he had some money, he could send freely for tickets to any cultural events that caught his eye: our regular theater series, Christmastime musicals, travel movies, folk artists.

Because he had some money he could look through tour brochures at pictures of Amsterdam, Naples, Marseilles, Vienna; and he could know that sometime we might really go.

Because he had some money I would find in his check register, at times when he was hospitalized and I was paying his bills, records of regular small donations: $25 to Disabled American Veterans who had assisted in his V.A. application, $30 to the Memphis State College scholarship fund, $20 to the local Association of Black Psychologists. I stared mesmerized at those mute statements of his wish to give, to give back. He had said to me years before, "I am not bitter," and he still was not. Not at all, not even a little bit. He was the opposite, appreciative and generous and more caring almost than his weak mute body could stand, and that was why he was able to be happy.

Generous especially with me, all his budding aching happiness circling itself around me. I was back to work and busy, but I came to see him almost every day. Something in me was still defensive about that, because of my own immersement in mental health taboos against too much giving, against martyrdom. But I wanted to come; these brief visits were the most rewarding hours of my days.

Harl welcomed me always with the same smile, already sitting in a spot on his sofa that left me room to slip in beside him. He kept a pillow there for me to support my head; I leaned back on it and turned to smile back at him, happiness flooding me as I had thought it could not do again. He listened raptly to my accounts of my days, fascinated with all the events of work or children or anything else going on with me. Or cried when I came in with pieces of a set of silverware I had bought at an antique store, because they were so pretty and because it was so unusual for me to do something like that for myself.

I read his newspaper, he sitting by me waiting for me to get to items he could point out to me. I pointed others out to him; we laughed or grimaced or shook our heads. Fighting back the ache of our silence, conversation of a sort, connecting at the intangible places where we were still soulmates.

No longer mindlessly watching whatever came on the television next, he studied the *TV Guide*, found the Arts and Entertainment channel and carefully mapped out his programs for a week. With cable many of those were delightfully in the daytime; he could get up and pour himself coffee and watch *African Queen* at nine in the morning.

He had been a man bone weary of working. I saw his contentment now and thought this release to delicious leisure might even be a reward.

But I was restless, always leaving finally, the pull of the world too strong for me. As I went I always went first to him, rubbing my cheek against his, nibbling at his ear. He smiled and made a sound like "Eah," watching me regretfully but forgivingly as I moved away. At the door I always turned back, finding it hard to separate. He leaned to see me and smiled again, waving goodbye; I smiled in our understanding of my own reluctance and waved back. Then I was out in the hall, the door closed behind me, heading back to that world of which he was no longer a part but I inextricably was.

* * *

Harl smiled and made his happy clapping gesture as I pushed open our motel room drapes, sunlight slanting across his face. We were vacationing for four days near San Diego. Though I had learned not to take him on any more two-week vacations, it was hard not to give him at least an occasional short trip. My spirits were not as good as his; time still dragged interminably.

He sat expectantly in his wheelchair, dressed neatly as always in a crisp light shirt and Bermuda shorts, ready for me to push him on our morning walk. I had been doing a lot of exploring of the area near our motel, walking for my therapy and even more to escape him.

It still seemed puzzling that being alone was not nearly the burden it was to be with someone who did not talk. It seemed I should be able to overcome my feelings about that silence, get to a place in my mind that made this confinement with Harl no worse than being alone. But I never could.

Our walk this morning was ambitious, I pushing the wheelchair to a beach near our motel. It was hard; there were hills, and I would not have tried it if I had not been so desperate. The walk gave us something to do to make the time pass, things I could talk to him about: the weather, houses we liked along the way, people on the beach. Inanities. My ability to talk this way always waned quickly; by evening I would be resorting to drinking too much, knocking myself out by nine o'clock to escape the silence. But Harl responded with animation, smiling and pointing himself. His knees below Bermuda shorts were knobby and unnaturally white, the pallor of one who rarely gets any sun. Below them his socks and laceup shoes were out of place, making my heart do one of its habitual painful twists. Should I have thought to take him shopping for summer shoes before we came here?

I was coming to terms with what Harl had called "non-nurturing" in me. I had lacked someone in my own life to cast an appraising eye over me and say, "Hey, we need to get you some shoes," or a haircut or whatever. I was not good at that with Harl or even with my children; they had to tell *me* when they needed things. It did not mean that I did not care, or that I would not give them or anyone the shirt off my back once the need was pointed out to me. It meant only that I did not notice. It was a trait.

At the beach I parked Harl's wheelchair under a palm tree and set off for my own daily walk by the ocean, relief welling with distance from him. At once the world was more vital, my own thoughts more entertaining.

I had dreamed. Harl was seeing a patient. His speech as he talked to her was not normal, but he could make himself understood. She had said something he was going to challenge; he leaned forward with his old look of shrewd wisdom, effortlessly finding just the right words to help her.

Though I had never actually seen Harl with a patient, I knew that was exactly how he would have looked. My first thought on waking had been that this was the first time since the stroke that I had allowed myself to dream of Harl as he was (and even now I had not let his speech be entirely normal). Until now such a dream would have been too painful to wake up from; that I could have it now must be a sign of my own healing.

That image of the old Harl stayed with me. I walked on the beach, looked at it in my mind and bade it a loving goodbye. The power, the competence, the gift of speech that made it all possible--those were gone, that Harl was gone.

He was replaced by the new Harl: gentle, easily

frightened, needing and accepting his need of me. I could dream of the old Harl now because I loved this new Harl too, probably more than the old. He was no less wise, and in spite of the loss of abstraction perhaps not really less intelligent. Only I knew how *much* knowledge was still trapped inside of him. I had slipped back into my old habit of asking him anything I wanted to know. Was Lyndon Johnson really drafting civil rights legislation while Jack Kennedy campaigned for president? (Yes.) Could there be such a thing as anti-gravity? (Probably.)

The waves rolled in and out; my feet made wet prints in the sand. I kept on. I was going to walk until this stretch of beach ended, and then I would go back to where Harl waited in his wheelchair under the tree. Waited with patience born of untold suffering, but waited knowing I would return. Knowing I would always return.

I looked back and saw that already my footprints were washing away. I saw too why that was such a common metaphor for time and loss. The pang I felt was because those footprints seemed a connection to Harl, vanishing like the talk we used to have.

The dream had prepared me for this wrench of loss. To have the conversation stripped from your love relationship is like an amputation. Like the sudden loss of an ear, only worse than that. Much worse than losing my ear.

So badly did I want him to talk to me just once more that I found a rock to sit on and hugged my own legs, resting my head on my knees. In a moment the anguish passed. It had been three years since he talked. You can get used to anything.

The ocean tugged at me, promising freedom and all the whispered joys of other worlds. But the little figure in the wheelchair tugged harder. My steps sped up as I headed back toward it. I rounded a bend and could see him, sitting just where I left him, watching the ocean and watching for me. He lit up when he saw me, but it would have been all right to wait a little longer too. That staggering patience had become his trademark. He was very strong.

*   *   *

Spring again. I came to him from work, kicking off my shoes to sit by him on his sofa. A breeze came through the balcony door, rustling art museum magazines on his coffee table.

I sat with a hand rested lightly on his leg and asked him what was the matter. He had been crying; when I asked why, he burst into tears again, pointing to a plaque he had laid on the table to show me. It was from the Rocky Mountain Psychological Association: *To Harl Henry Young, Distinguished Service Award.*

An old friend or acquaintance from the Association had brought it by. Harl talked and gestured, showing me how the two of them had sat awhile on his balcony. He said resolutely, "And I didn't dry duh whole time!"

But as soon as the person left, he had sat down and cried the rest of the afternoon. I asked him what time that was; he said, "About dree o'tlock."

It was six now. He had been crying for three hours.

So they did remember him. I stared wordless at the plaque.

Another day at my house he cried not in his usual easy way but setting his teeth against the tears, pointing to a newspaper headline: *Mentally Ill Homeless.* His fist clenched in one anguished helpless gesture. *Harl Henry Young* had emptied out the State Hospital, wielding his immense personal power to create a community based mental health system. A model system, one of the nation's first. His publications in that area were vast; he had been a national leader and authority; after twenty years many other systems were still modeled on his. How could he have imagined how ruthlessly State legislatures would gnaw away the financial base for the community systems, the treatment centers, the halfway houses. The social supports, the food. *Mentally Ill Homeless.* Harl had done what he set out to do, made the mental health delivery system more humane. And over the next decade, that humanity had been taken away.

* * *

Everyone in his building spoke to Harl. He had made himself again a person of consequence, someone noticed and remembered. In stores eyes lingered on him as he passed. Therapists adored him and came to see him at home if he could not get out; cleaning people liked him so much they reduce their rates to come more often.

He did it with his smile. It was a smile of such simple radiance as to stun people into momentary suspension, then leave them feeling oddly better. I grew used to hearing it commented upon: "He has such a beautiful smile!"

A record club must have sent him an advertisement. He bought himself a radio/tape deck, and after that I seldom found him watching television anymore. He suddenly had tapes, classical pieces carefully chosen. I would come from work and find him seated dreamily on the sofa, the balcony door open to let in the breeze, waving his arms as if conducting the orchestra. On seeing me, he would start to smile, then often break instead into unexpected tears at the sheer beauty of it all: his apartment, the music, me coming in.

He beamed on me, sitting close to put a hand on mine. I said something about being sorry he did not have more visitors, and he said he did not need other visitors because he had me. He gestured around him at the room and the music and me, and said he had enough.

The most extraordinary experience I could ever have, going to Harl in his apartment and seeing that smile he gave me.

Perhaps it was out of his Southern roots that he had the special love he did for Gospel music, but I thought it was also because it was a music with so much depth to it. Meeting me one evening extra eager for me to hear his newest tape, he limped to the stereo to put it on; then had to stop with a hand to his mouth as Paul Robeson sang out in rich baritone, *Swing Low Sweet Chariot*.

Yet he startled me by saying a few minutes later that he would not especially mind dying. I felt a shadow of anxiety, looked at him and said I had thought he was happy? He said he was happy. But still....

He explained, gesturing to his balcony and out toward the city beyond it. He sat on his balcony, he said, and looked out over the city and thought about all the life that was going on out there, all the people busy doing things with each other. "And I miss dat. So I don't mind dying so mutz."

I could have felt the crunch of failure that for all my effort I had not been able to keep him from that. But his own rich quiet smile stopped me. We were separate people after all; it was not possible for me to fill up so much loss. I touched his face, warm in the hollow I loved, and struggled for my own acceptance. I had given him all I could give, and he gave back all he could give, but still...

Still, he would not mind dying so much.

I would mind. His heart was not good; the time could not be that far off. Even now I had to get myself ready, look around this place of so much hard won happiness and imagine that one day I would come for a last time to it, and he would not be in it. The door would be open just like that, the breeze rustling the same magazines, all his books and papers in the same impeccable order. But there would be no smile, no love to welcome me.

I had to keep making myself ready.

* * *

On an Easter Sunday we went to a service at an Episcopal Church. There were flowers and rousing music; Harl beamed happily beside me. The sermon was about crucifixion and resurrection, how the true meaning of Easter is that after crucifixion there is always resurrection. Even now my skeptical mind thought of the less fortunate population of the world and questioned that *always*. But Harl and I were not starving in the Third World; for us there had been opportunity, and we had taken it and made our resurrection.

That afternoon as we lay on my bed Harl touched me and said, without tears this time, "I have never been happier in my whole life."

EPILOGUE

I

Who will sing
for me?
   --"Who Will Sing For Me?"

    The end began on a night at my house after dinner and theatre. We had made love, not just with our hands as we usually did but really making love. Every once in a while Harl could do that, and it always made him happy. I fell asleep with his heart racing under my hand, the lurching shallow thuds that were normal for him, that told me as always how fragile this happiness we had still was.
    He had got up early to use the bathroom; I lay with eyes still closed listening for the limping sound of his return. He settled back in beside me.
    And in the next second was reeled back on the pillow gasping like a fish. I was up with a half scream, first reaching for him in a confused futile attempt to help, then seizing the phone to call an ambulance. "This is a heart patient and he's having some kind of attack. I think he's dying; they have to come *quick*."
    How quick would quick be? He had turned blue and could make no sound except that terrible gasping. He stared at me, beseeching and yet with a gentleness so profound that even in the midst of this I wondered at it. *Infinitely gentle, infinitely suffering.* His head went back, and his throat

rattled.

I thought the rattle meant he was dying right then, but somehow he didn't. He kept on gasping, and looking at me with that mute beseeching gentleness, and then the ambulance people were in the room.

There was not time to take him to the hospital where Dr. Friedman practiced; they had to get him to whatever hospital was nearest. As they moved him to a stretcher, his gasping faded and his eyes rolled back. One of them drove a fist into his chest, and he started gasping again.

People swarmed around him in the emergency room, giving him oxygen, suctioning his lungs. He had never lost consciousness; he lay with eyes comprehending and kept on gasping. I watched from the back of the room, out of everyone's way. I had not seen real heart failure before; I had no idea how horrible it was.

A doctor pulled me out to the hallway to talk. I told him about the plastic heart valve, the stroke, the other more minor episodes of congestive heart failure.

He said, "He is probably not going to pull through this. My best guess is that the valve has torn loose. If that is the case, will you want us to replace it again?"

Rephrase: Is his life worth that much suffering to him to save? I could not be having to make this decision at such a time, my eye blink rate at near zero from my own shock. I asked numbly, "Could he survive the surgery?" and noted the small fleeting part of me that wanted the answer I got.

"That is very unlikely. I have to tell you I think he would not survive it."

I said, "Then don't do it," and went back and stared at Harl where he still lay gasping, and wondered if I had just killed him.

Cathryn found us upstairs in the cardiac intensive care

unit. Harl was somehow still alive, hooked to I.V.s, a respirator tube now down his throat. I had assumed a right to stay in this room with him; I thought that after talking for him for so long, I was like a part of him. So far no one had challenged me. I stayed inconspicuously in a chair in a corner, a blanket hiding the turning of my shock to chills.

Cathryn and I went out in the hall to talk. She was seventeen; I was to be taking her for college interviews in just two weeks. She had lived with a lot with Harl's stroke and so much of my attention diverted to him, and then my illness, and now this. Her hand touched mine; she asked, "Are you going to be all right, Mom?"

I said I would be all right. I said this had been coming for a long time, and I would be all right. But I wanted to stay. Would she bring me my toothbrush and address book?

I wrapped up in my blanket again, and David walked in. Cathryn had called him; he said she had been crying. We went to the hall again. David had gone from eighteen to twenty-two while I hardly noticed. He put an arm around my shoulders and said, "You'll be all right, Mom."

The doctors no longer thought the valve had come loose. But they still thought Harl would not make it. Dopamine dripping through the I.V.s was all that kept his heart beating, and the respirator with the tube down his throat was all that kept his lungs going. Whatever part of me had thought fleetingly that I was ready to be released from him was quite gone; I shivered in my corner and could not take my eyes off him.

Steve and Cathryn came with the toothbrush and address book, and a change of clothes, and books to read. The three of us went to dinner in the cafeteria, letting the nurses know so they could get me on short notice. Steve was awkward, Cathryn depressed. After they left I went back and sat reading in Harl's room, surprised that I could even now escape that way.

When he moved or moaned, I went to him. He stared beseechingly at me; he wanted me to get the tube out of his throat. His look was not at all the gentle surprised expression of that morning, but hopeless now, despairing. When I failed to help him, his eyes turned to the ceiling, and his shackled hand made a movement of hopeless futility.

Was there any way to make the tube more comfortable? It seemed to be pressing painfully on his tongue, but the nurses said that could not be helped. They would alternate it at the next shift with one that went through his nose, but that kind was just as bad.

Just as I used to call Senior Wheels at four fifty-five because after five I would not be able to call them, now as eight and then nine at night approached, the pressure inside me to *do something* grew stronger. I questioned the nurse, feeling my words come as if from a great distance. "Is it really any use keeping him on that respirator when it makes him suffer so much? Don't the doctors think he's going to die anyway?"

She said at once, "If you want the respirator discontinued, you can call and talk to Dr.____. Probably the better thing to do if we were going to do that would be to stop the Dopamine."

She had not said those things should not be done.

That mounting inside pressure made me pace. I went from one end of the hall to the other and back, then again, and then pushed open a door to a stairwell and after it another marked For Emergency Use Only, and found myself on a fire escape.

The bars were cool; I sat and leaned my face against them. Below me in the dark was the city, heedless as ever of my own small universe. Harl and Bonnie, Bonnie and Harl. With the stroke I had already been through so much with him. It seemed unfair that I should also have to do this, make this decision that was not even related to the stroke.

Except that it was, of course. The quality of life questions were about the stroke, and that I had never talked to Harl about a living will was because of the stroke. I had known he needed one but thought he was too emotional and could not deal with it. And of course I had not imagined a thing like this, his landing in a strange hospital away from his own doctors.

But everything, always, was because of the stroke.

It was past nine; if I wanted to spare Harl having that tube down his throat the whole night, I would have to act soon. But I wasn't ready to call Dr. _____, because I didn't know what to ask for, and because I didn't know what to do if he said no.

That was what I expected. It was the kind of story that was in the newspapers all the time. Families go to court trying to stop a respirator; an elderly husband shoots his wife in her hospital bed. And this was a Seventh Day Adventist hospital; they didn't even have meat in the cafeteria. Would they discontinue life supports?

What would I do if they would not take the tube out? My mind raced, crafty, criminal. They did sometimes leave me in Harl's room alone with him. But with all the monitors he was on, there would be no way I could tamper with the oxygen or the I.V.s without someone's being alerted. I had no idea how to get hold of a syringe or a lethal dose of something. I had no idea even what a lethal dose of anything was.

I shut my eyes, pressed my face harder against the bars and felt the pressure inside me melting into fear. The only way to do it would be openly. Buy a gun, walk in and shoot him. The fear that made my breath ragged came from my sense of my own rather high potential for doing such a thing.

Harl had said of Dian, *If it hadn't been for the possibility of criminal charges.* He was more humble than I; compassion in me intersected dangerously with my contempt for inhumane authority. *They had no right.*

But they did have the power, and that was what Harl had the humility to know. I could not risk the criminal charges, even for him. Even to get that tube out of his throat, to respond to his beseeching hopeless look, his turning of his eyes in that terrible despair to the ceiling. Even though I was his voice, and he totally dependent on me. It was beyond what one person could do for another; it was not to be considered.

The nurse had said I could call Dr. ____. I went back inside and first called Dr. Friedman, reaching Neil. I had already talked to both Neil and Dr. Friedman several times today, and Neil had come by late in the afternoon. But the doctors here were not welcoming their involvement; Dr. Friedman told me they felt they had to stay out of it.

Why did my words sound so tentative to me, when actually they were quite to the point? It was because there was so much feeling under them that went unspoken.

"Harl is suffering so much on the respirator, and the doctors have said they don't think he'll live. Is it reasonable to be keeping him on it?"

An intake of breath, like a murmured *oh* as Neil realized what I was asking. He said he would want Dr. Friedman to call me about that. But he did know what I meant: "As long as Harl has been coming here, he has always had his spirit. We've never seen him like this, the way he looks up at the ceiling in that complete despair."

I waited in the pay phone booth, jumping at the ring that

came almost at once. Dr. Friedman was very gentle, very caring. "We don't know enough about his condition right now to tell you what we would recommend. You will have to talk about that with Dr. _____. I can tell you though that if Harl does pull through this, it is likely that in another couple of months he will be back with something similar.

"We know what it was to Harl to lose his speech"--even now tears rolled onto my cheeks on hearing those words; horror still said *No, nothing that bad could happen to Harl*-- "and how he has struggled since then, and what you have been to him. Our prayers are with you."

I went back and stood by Harl again, rubbing his curled right hand. Oxygen deprivation during the heart failure must have worsened his stroke symptoms; the hand lay as helpless as when the stroke first happened. Again his eyes beseeched me, then turned to the ceiling as his left hand moved in that same helpless hopeless gesture.

I went back to the phone booth and called Dr. _____. He was not particularly nice. But he did indicate they would disconnect the respirator if that was my request. I remembered then that downstairs across from the cafeteria there was a rack with forms for Living Wills. Apparently this hospital had a different policy than those of the newspaper stories. They would stop the respirator if I asked.

But he did not recommend it. He sounded affronted, as if I were a nuisance or a bad person, as if my question was out of line. "There is nothing in this chart that would make *me* think we should give up now."

He was a night doctor and had not even seen Harl, but he did have the chart. I could not say to stop the life supports if the doctor thought there was hope.

From my chair in the corner I stared at Harl or out the window into the darkness. Finally I grew tired enough to take my blanket to a deserted waiting room down the hall, telling the nurse, "Please get me if *anything* happens." She promised she would; she said she understood.

Understood what? I did not understand myself. I lay on a sofa gazing unseeingly at a flickering television across the room and wondered at my own single consuming wish, which was to be with him when he died. I had talked for him for so long; he must be less frightened with me there. And we were so close, so close. I was his voice, he was my--

He was my heart.

The nurse never called me, but I woke in the dark early morning hours anyway. Harl slept fitfully now, blessedly dopey on medication. When the first sun came through the window, he was still alive.

Cathryn brought me shampoo and a towel. I ducked my head under the cold water of the tiny bathroom on Harl's floor, furtive as if I were doing something criminal. Probably visitors were not supposed to use these bathrooms for washing their hair.

Wet-headed, I went outside with Cathryn to walk in the sun. She wore thongs and cutoffs. Her legs were slender and deep brown; the sun hit every gold highlight in her hair. We went to the cafeteria and ate boiled eggs and toast and coffee. She left and I went back to Harl, carrying another cup of coffee with me. A doctor was there, the one who had first told me Harl would probably not live through this. He said Harl's signs were looking a little better. They would try cutting back some on the Dopamine and see if he could keep his blood pressure up without it.

And they would see if he could manage on nasal oxygen instead of the respirator.

A nurse came to pull the tube out. Harl's body convulsed and he made a gagging sound as she did it, and then it was out and he took a tremendous relieved breath, and looked at her and smiled his beautiful warm smile.

I stretched my arm around him and laid my cheek in the hollow of his cheek and neck, and laughed and wept at the same time as he reached for my hand and turned that same smile on me.

Four years of progress with the stroke had been wiped out, at least temporarily. Just days before, I had been thinking how perfect Harl's notes had become; frustrating as it was for him not to be able to speak intelligibly, he could always communicate if he had to by writing a note. Now he could no longer spell my name, or write an intelligible sentence.

Hopefully some of this would pass as brain swelling went down. He was moved to a rehabilitation unit, where he started counting the days until he could go home. I came by every day after work, but it was hard now to visit him. How does one pass the time in a hospital room with a patient who cannot talk? I ran through my news from the day, about work, about Cathryn's college applications.

Usually I ended by just lying down on Harl's bed beside him, where I could put an arm across his chest and rest my head on his shoulder. Sometimes I even slept.

Sometimes a nurse or doctor came in, and I moved back guiltily wondering if they would tell me to stay off the bed. Lying on beds with patients probably wasn't proper.

When Harl wanted to go home, he meant *home*; his own apartment, not my house where I offered to keep him until he was stronger. He shook his head eagerly, and pronounced the word as he always did, happily, with an oddly heavy accent on the second syllable: "My t'a*paht*ment!"

I took him there. He sank onto his sofa and looked slowly around, at the pictures, the desk with his many piles of papers, the books in their dark bookcases, the table with the peach color in its cloth, the balcony with the view beyond it stretching over the city. Peace and relief flooded his face. Finally he smiled back over at me, and asked me to make us some drinks.

* * *

The pile of mail waiting for him included an announcement of a psychological convention in Moscow: "The Year of the Child," sponsored jointly by Russian and American psychological associations. Harl had not been home even a week when we signed up.

Dr. Friedman was not crazy about the idea. But Harl was just that, crazy about it. He tapped my arm as we sat in Ray and Virginia's living room, saying eagerly, "Tell dem d'about Wussia!" and smiled radiantly and moved his fist in a cheering gesture when I did.

Ray and Virginia asked me privately if I had thought how awful it would be for me if he died over there. I replied fatalistically that it was Harl's choice to live as fully as he could. I would not stop him from doing anything his doctors did not absolutely prohibit.

Two weeks before the October trip, I found him lying panting on his sofa. He tried to smile to reassure me, laying a hand gently on my shoulder as I bent over him. He started to say no as I said I would call an ambulance, then seemed to see I must do it. As I hung up he said, "I'm dorry d'about *Wussia*." And as I leaned down to hold him again he added hopefully, "Maybe *dyou* tan dill doe."

I hugged him and told him I would not go to Russia without him.

He had been driving, on his way to the grocery store and dry cleaner, when he began to breathe this way. He had turned around and come home, parked his car and got himself upstairs and into his apartment. That had been hours ago; he had been lying here like this most of the afternoon. Resting my hands on either side of his chest, I asked him why he had not pushed the emergency button on his Lifeline. Or at least speed dialed me at my office. He looked surprised; he answered simply, "I knew wen dyou tame, dyou would know wat to do."

This time the doctors diagnosed progressive lung disease, *pulmonary fibrosis*. Heart failure and lung failure worked against each other, each making the other worse.

Harl would have to be put on continuous oxygen. He would need a stationary tank for his apartment and a portable one with a cart for when he went out.

He wanted only to go to Russia. All the doctors who examined him at the hospital knew it. They would talk to him about his echocardiogram or his blood oxygen levels, and he would answer, "Tan I doe to *Wussia*?"

Dr. Friedman said he could not in good conscience write a letter saying Harl was safe to fly, but the staff cardiologist would. His attitude was more like mine: "This man just really wants to go to Russia!"

Armed with the letter, I talked to the tour company. Passengers were not allowed to bring their own oxygen onto aircrafts, but we could get oxygen arranged on the domestic flights and on Air Lingus to Ireland. But from Shannon we were taking the Russian Aero Flot to Moscow. Aero Flot could be reached only by telegram from the Shannon airport, and they kept telegraphing back, "This man will not be permitted to board."

Harl greeted me each day bursting with hope and

suspense. The tour company wanted me to give it up, but I looked at Harl and stifled the small voice inside me that said they were right, and went at it again. I was trying to get Aero Flot to reconsider, and also find out how to get portable oxygen in Russia. Russians must get pulmonary fibrosis too; didn't they have oxygen suppliers?

At two a.m. my time I spoke with the pleasant heartily-brogued director of the Shannon Airport, who said cheerfully that in twenty years he had never heard of such a thing but he would send Aero Flot another telegram. Dozens of times through several nights I dialed the U.S. Embassy in Moscow, but the only time there was an answer it was a janitor who said no one was in.

It was ten a.m. there. What time did they come in? He said he didn't know.

Harl was having to miss a wedding in which I was the maid of honor. I came to the hospital after it in my burgundy bridesmaid's dress, the broad-brimmed matching hat still on my head, to share as much as I could of it with him. He cried when he saw me, one hand to his mouth, the other gesturing up and down me as he said, "Dyou d'yook doe bootiful!"

Back home, I continued my middle of the night phone calls.

At least Harl knew I had given it everything I had. We were like conspirators alone together in the world, Us against Them. I flopped beside him on his bed one day before his discharge and three before we were to have left on our trip, and told him the thing could not be done.

He was not devastated. Disappointed, but realistically so. He took my hand with a resigned but still beautifully warm smile and said, "I d'yuv you."

The stationary oxygen tank was waiting in his apartment, with a sound like the breathing of a great beast. I felt myself look at it a little sideways, as if to avoid the full impact of it. Harl was to spend the rest of his life leashed to that thing?

His tubing trailed behind him as he moved about the room. I had thought with his concrete thinking he would be really depressed by this, but he seemed less affected than I. Maybe because he had not accepted it; I would learn shortly that he had every intention of going out without the oxygen as he pleased, as always.

The portable tanks were cumbersome. I had talked with the supplier and chosen an electric oxygenator rather than liquid oxygen with lighter portable units, because the electric unit could be taken to my house. The stationary liquid unit was too heavy to move, and the portable component would not last long enough to get Harl through a night. I asked about getting him two or three of the portable liquid components; that would not work because they leaked and still might not get him through a night.

So the plug-in oxygenator that could with some difficulty be hauled over to my house was all that kept Harl, except for brief excursions with the portable tanks, from being permanently chained to his home. Hiding my own depression, I rolled the thing to the elevator and lifted it into my car that very first night. We were going to dinner and then to my house. Harl would not live chained like an animal in thirty feet of space.

* * *

One night after dinner at his apartment Harl motioned to me to stay, returning to the sofa and pulling out what explained the secret happiness I had sensed in him this whole evening. It was December, and what he had were advertisements from jewelry stores. He wanted to buy me a diamond ring for Christmas.

I had never had a diamond. When my friends in college were all absorbed with diamonds, I had not understood it. I had married on a student budget and not given a ring a thought; I thought my friends with their craze for diamond rings were being materialistic.

The *cherishing* meaning in diamonds had gone quite by me, because I could not imagine myself being cherished.

Harl pointed to different pictures, rings seeming to shoot light, gorgeously displayed. His face was rich with happiness; I had never seen anything mean more to him than this.

We went on a snowy evening to the jewelry store, I wheeling his oxygen behind him, holding his arm so he would not slip. He sat by me as the jeweler pulled rings from a case, studying them on my finger, smiling yes or shaking his head no. His eyes brimmed from time to time with happy tears. I worried about price, but Harl waved his hand to say that was not a concern. He picked the most gorgeous of all the rings I had tried on, tears brimming again through his smile as his motion said that was his favorite. He gestured manfully to the jeweler, pulling out his credit cards.

Harl teased me with the ring, saying I could not have it until Christmas but could look at it at his apartment. Now each day I found him staring at it, looking up with joy to hold it out to me as I came in. He must have spent hours with it, turning it in the light, smiling or crying over it. It gleamed at me from its dark box; I said it was the most beautiful thing I had ever seen.

He let me wear it while I was there, making me take it off before I left. Until Christmas, when I sat by him under the tree at my house and slid it on and pressed my lips to the warm curve of his neck, and called it my *permanently engaged* ring.

*   *   *

There was still that persistent small part of me that sometimes thought it wanted the release that only Harl's death would bring. But it vanished any time I arrived at his apartment and did not find him immediately in sight. Then my heart lurched as I called out, "Harl?"

On hearing him answer, "Eah!" from the kitchen or bedroom, I took deep breaths of relief.

My wish to be with him when he died seemed unlikely to be granted me. Given that we spent many more hours apart than together, it was more likely I would come one day and find him as I feared each of those times I did not see him right away. Unless he grew ill with enough warning to be in a hospital, and then there would be the nightmare of needles in him and a tube down his throat. I did not know which would be worse. I just wanted to be with him.

Harl kept showing me the travel brochures that came regularly to his apartment: Florence, Amsterdam, the South of France. Cruises seemed promising, a way for him to travel while still staying in one place. I called on some of those, but they would not let him have oxygen on the ships.

And everything was so expensive, four thousand dollars for a vacation while I had three children in college. I told Harl we would find something eventually that I could afford.

We took shorter trips, a visit to Cindy in Albany and an Amtrak ride from there to Manhattan for a day, and then on to Richmond for some days with Robin. Or a flight to Ottawa for a weekend with an old friend of Harl's who had seen him with me at a psychology meeting, and alone out of that whole mental health community wrote and asked him to visit.

* * *

He was in the hospital again, oddly for the fourth October since his stroke. The only October that he had missed being hospitalized was in the year of my surgery.

This time the doctors were looking more at the lung disease. His oxygen requirement had doubled in a year, from two liters a minute to four. At that level the nasal canula began to be inefficient; more oxygen blew off than came through.

More than anything else, more than the stroke even, this relentless progressing lung disease made me sick at heart. It was the worst way to die; he was going to suffer so much. Better to drop with a heart attack, better even for me to have to find him. I talked in the hall with Dr. Friedman, feeling that just an explanation would make me feel better. Harl had quit smoking before his first heart surgery ten years before and never touched a cigarette since. And there had been no hint of lung disease then.

I asked, "Don't you have some idea what is causing the lung disease? And why is it progressing so rapidly?"

Dr. Friedman repeated what he had told me many times already. The pulmonary fibrosis was of unknown origin, possibly linked in some way to repeated episodes of congestive heart failure. There was no way known to medicine to slow it down.

He said sadly, "What Harl should really have is a heart

transplant. Or in his case a heart and lung transplant. Heart transplants have become the most frequently performed surgery at University Hospital. But they won't take a patient with anything else wrong with him, so the stroke would rule Harl out."

The thought of it made me a little giddy, Harl with a healthy heart and lungs, no more gray-blue hands and face, no more pausing to pant after walking a few yards. It could be done.

But not for him, because of the stroke. Dr. Friedman was telling me instead about a new procedure for providing oxygen trans-tracheally, through a tube surgically implanted into the throat. It was actually less visible and more pleasant to wear than the nasal canulas, and because there was no blow-off, it permitted the litre flow to be increased indefinitely. He strongly recommended it.

This would mean Harl could no longer go out as he liked to do for a couple of hours without his oxygen. He would be really chained to it now, carting it with him everywhere he went for the rest of his life. I still cringed from that, but Dr. Friedman said that by now he should not be going without the oxygen even for those short stretches anyway. The trans-tracheal delivery was a real breakthrough and would make him much more comfortable.

Harl sat back weakly on his pillows, his hands black and blue from blood tests and I.V.s. He was calculating how soon they would let him out. He had gone in on a Tuesday and thought they would probably not let him go before the weekend. So his hopes were pinned on Monday.

As before, I passed my visits with him by climbing onto the bed and resting with an arm around him. A pulmonary doctor had been in to talk to him about the trans-tracheal oxygen procedure. Harl tried to tell me about it, pointing to

his throat and saying, "Button."
And he wrote:

> He a surgeon ~~over~~ compound
> 2 services, surgeon also.
> He's told about a machine
> which ~~we~~ gereate as long
> in a place. Then you
> move it and it performs
> the same way. If it
> likes it, maybe I can
> ~~get~~ take with us.

I told him Dr. Friedman thought it was a really good idea. He said with uncommon excitement for any medical procedure, "Den dyet's do it!"

It was an outpatient surgery, first insertion of a temporary tube and two weeks later the permanent one. He was switched after the first visit to liquid oxygen, with a plastic portable unit that weighed only two pounds. Now that he had to take it with him everywhere, he had to have the lighter units.

Since trans-tracheally he could use a lower litre flow, he would still be able to spend nights at my house. I would keep some compressed tanks there too, to hook him to the next day so he could also spend Sunday mornings.

I had to do all that figuring for myself because no one else understood how important those nights and mornings at my house were. Anyone else would naturally think that I could just go stay at Harl's place instead. But that was not even close to as good, because it was so confining for him and also because I had no way to pass the time there. At my house I could keep getting up and doing things, get some cooking started, clean a little, wash my hair. Between activities I came back to bed, made Harl another Bloody Mary, talked a little until I fizzled out again from the one-sidedness of conversation. Often we kept that up until one or two in the afternoon.

Whereas at Harl's place I was frantic by nine o'clock.

After the second visit when they inserted the permanent tube, the technician asked if we still had any questions. We had been shown films about the care of the catheter, and Harl had practiced cleaning it while she watched. I said I didn't think I had any questions.

We both looked at Harl, crisp as always in a white shirt and blue and white striped sports jacket. He pointed to the oxygen tank in its aluminum cart and asked, "Wen do I det wid of dat?"

Whatever could he mean? Foreboding blew over me like a chilly wind.

The technician thought he was asking to have the procedure reversed. She said, "I thought we told you this was permanent. Once it's done, it isn't usually reversed." He pointed more persistently at the tank, beginning to look dismayed. "But wen do I det wid of *dat*?"

She said again that the procedure was permanent. He pointed then to his throat and said, "Button!"

Understanding better than she but wishing I didn't, I broke in. "Harl." He looked at me. I asked, "Did you think you weren't going to have the tanks anymore?"

He nodded vigorously, excited. Perhaps since I understood, I could help him. He said insistently again, "*Button*," pointing to the small piece of clear plastic that was like a button at his throat, where the catheter went in.

I said, "But you have to have the tank. It's where your oxygen comes from."

He crumpled suddenly, weeping in long slow despairing sobs. Just once more he lifted his head to turn and appeal to me, wailing, "*Button!*"

I saw how it had happened. So much conversation went by him; even the doctors did not know as I did how to get his attention. Always I started a sentence twice, or said his name and then paused before starting. Trying to follow as the doctor explained this to him, he had seized on that one word, *button*, and somehow imagined his oxygen would be miraculously delivered by a button pushed at his throat. No more tubes, no more tanks to haul around, freedom. How many times had I had this thought that I could not stand to see him disappointed again?

He cried so hard, yet by the next day he had rallied again. Everywhere he went now he pushed his oxygen cart in front of him, without apology, without complaint. Still smiling his old smile, still Harl.

* * *

Carolyn at the hospital called and said Medicare would not pay for his speech therapy anymore. "We've really kept him longer than we should have already, because we loved him so. He isn't improving anymore; we can't justify it."

Another door closing. I said I hated to see it end because it was something for him to do. "He talks to you, he likes you. It's the only place he goes."

She had an idea. There was an aphasia group that met Wednesday mornings at the Washington Park Community Center right in our neighborhood. "Sometimes they have parties or go places together. I know last month they went to a matinee down at Stage West. If you'd like, I'll call the speech therapist who leads it and talk to her about Harl."

I told her to talk to Harl about it first. This sounded hopeful. Maybe if I went with him the first few times, he would warm up to it.

He surprised me. He had carefully written down the information Carolyn gave him and wanted very much to go. He pulled it out as soon as I arrived, pointing to the dates, asking eagerly if I could go to just the first meeting with him, "To det me *tarted.*"

I met him there, turning my staff meeting over to Bonnie H., arriving at ten-fifteen for the ten-thirty group to be sure Harl would not have to meet them the first time alone. His car pulled up right behind mine; he got out with the happy look he always had for me.

There were fifteen or twenty of them, mostly men, a few with wives. All talked better than Harl, but all were impaired. They watched us from around the table with naked fascination, struggling for words, crippled arms drawn up.

All of them were so sweet. I thought fleetingly of the Little Prince coming on a whole garden of roses, when he had thought his own loved rose was the only one.

One of them succeeded in asking, "What was he?"

I told them, speaking proudly for him. "He was a *psychologist*. He taught at the University of Denver."

Another said, "Who are you?"

I answered proudly again, taking his hand. "I'm his girlfriend."

* * *

December came cold and bright, with so far just a few light snowfalls. Harl stayed in with any snowfall at all, turning on his music, thumbing through the mail order arrivals at his apartment: museum bulletins, travel brochures, food and wine magazines. Treasures of the world in picture form.

We looked from the warmth of his apartment through the balcony windows to the blowing December snow, and both shuddered. He was weaker than he used to be, and slower. Getting to and from our car and a restaurant or theater was harder, because we got so cold. I said I thought it was time we got him a wheelchair.

I knew it was hard for someone fighting decline to accept a wheelchair, so I made as light of it as I could. "Not for all the time, but so you can go more places. I could take you downtown on Saturdays, and we could walk up and down the mall and look at the Christmas decorations."

His eyes clicked into the thoughtful internal look that meant he was not just jumping at my fantasy but considering something beneath the surface of it. He smiled gently then and said with a nod but also a touch of resignation, "I dink I would d'yike a weeltair now."

If Medicare didn't pay for it, the insurance I still carried on Harl through my company probably would.

A morning of phone calls as Harl sat beside me in my bed with his Bloody Mary, and I had found the best one. We drove to the medical supply house to look at it. They called it a sports model, and it was so different from other wheelchairs that it made us laugh: red and black, with padded over-sized wheels for a smooth ride, eight pounds lighter than the other lightest wheelchair made. *Spiffy*. And it had been used on the floor for demonstrations and so was on sale; Medicare would not pay for extra-light chairs, but this one cost no more than an ordinary chair.

Harl sat in it, laying his cane smartly across the arm rests. A clerk showed me how to hang his oxygen tank between the handle bars behind him. I wheeled him once around the shop, and he clapped and waved happily for me to go ahead and buy it. He had some money; he could get this very special chair even if none of his insurance paid.

I pushed him on out through the cold to the car, his cane still smartly across the arm rests, oxygen hanging down behind him, white canvas cap pulled low over his forehead. Happiness filled me like a helium balloon.

When I was younger, a teenager or young wife and mother, even in the early years of living with Harl, I had thought happiness was something very different from this. How could I get this happy, over buying a wheelchair?

* * *

Through the winter and spring Harl went faithfully every Wednesday morning to his aphasia group, staying at the Center for a potluck lunch and a movie in the afternoons.

Sometimes the group had a picnic or a trip to a museum; then I took off work and went with him, pushing him in his spiffy red wheelchair. But the best thing about the group was that it was a place Harl could go without me, and be with other people.

My business had picked up again, miraculously undiminished by the law change. Now we did vocational evaluations to determine injured workers' loss of earning capacity, and the demand for those evaluations was increasing. Superstitious about believing in good things because then they would probably go away, I nevertheless finally told Harl one afternoon as I slid in beside him on his sofa that I was starting to feel secure again.

Except about him, about his lungs. But I did not tell him that. In just eight months since he went on the trans-tracheal oxygen, his litre flow had doubled. I had stopped fearing he would die suddenly in heart failure; I knew he was going to die slowly and horribly from the lung disease. He would be institutionalized, the one thing in the world that sent him into abject helpless weeping. He would be hooked interminably to machines.

Wondering if perhaps he knew more of this than he let on, I told him that if there were times when he needed extra care, we would have him come stay again with me. I had thought about that and knew it would be hard for me, but I would do it to keep him from an institution. I pictured him in my bed hooked to oxygen and I.V.s, probably with a nurse for while I was at work. He would smile weakly at me when I came home; he would be there warm beside me reading or watching television in the evenings. I would bring him things, help him to the bathroom, care for him.

Harl looked dismayed. Apparently he really had not thought about any of this. He looked around him at his apartment and said in deep anxiety that he wanted to stay there.

I said maybe it wouldn't happen. But that I wanted him to know he could stay with me if he needed to.

* * *

My new Visa Gold Card had come with a blurb about special cardholder benefits, among them assistance with medical needs while traveling. I had first used their assistance center when Harl and I missed a connection on one of our many short trips, leaving him stranded without oxygen. Now they were getting his oxygen arranged for the vacation we were finally planning for the next October, in Costa Rica.

They called me several times a week, making sure I had the right doctor letters, making sure the airlines had their orders right. Dr. Friedman was not entirely comfortable writing a letter saying Harl was safe to fly, but his pulmonary doctor was. So I worked with him about what the letter and prescription should say. I was anxious that they absolutely match; any confusion and an airline would put us off.

Harl was to get his oxygen while flying at four liters a minute. Most airlines offered either two or four, with four costing twice as much as two. But one of them had a different kind of bottle and could provide only two or three. I talked by phone with Dr. Christopher; he said three would be all right.

Because I had become experienced at this, I asked him to provide a range. So he said two to four, as needed. The letter we were to carry with us also said it would be more comfortable for Harl if he could hook the airline's equipment to his trans-tracheal tube. Weeks before the trip, because I was so afraid of forgetting it, I tucked an extra plastic connecting piece into my purse so that the airline's tubing could be hooked to his trans-tracheal tube.

It would not have surprised me at all if an airline put us off just because they didn't understand the trans-tracheal equipment. We had been put off before over small differences between the letter the doctor wrote for us and the prescription he wrote for them.

I loved the Visa people. They called everyone over and over, to make sure nothing went wrong. Their representative in Costa Rica was arranging the oxygen for our hotel, and would meet us at the San Jose airport. So would someone from the medical supply company, with a portable tank to get Harl to the hotel. And so would someone from the tour company that had booked our trip. We would be met by a veritable entourage.

What else could go wrong? I asked the Visa people to make sure the person from the medical supplier would come into the hotel with us, so we would know the equipment there was working before he or she left us. We were promised that person would speak English.

Suppliers in Atlanta and Miami were meeting us with oxygen for our layovers. The Visa people called them over and over too, double and triple checking the orders, making sure nothing was misunderstood. They called me several times to make sure I had the names and phone numbers of those suppliers, so I could reach them quickly if anything got screwed up.

I loved the Visa people because they shared my understanding that things always got screwed up.

Airlines never accepted advance payment on the oxygen; Harl had to pay for that at the ticket counters just before departure. This was nerve-wracking if we were changing airlines and did not have long layovers, but this time our layovers were two to three hours, so it did not look like a problem.

I ran down my mind like a checklist. What else could go wrong? We were taking Harl's own wheelchair and needed it for the layovers. The Visa people verified several times with each airline that the chair could be cabin checked.

Harl who still had difficulty reading had read all the Costa Rica guidebooks, including sections on political history. Each evening as I arrived at his apartment he pulled them out, pointing to special sections he had marked for me, his smile spilling over me. I was getting our day tours arranged in advance, to make sure there would not be unexpected problems with the oxygen or wheelchair. Harl had found us a day trip to the beach at Punta Reynas, and we were going to the Poas National Park cloud forest "with thirty-eight species of birdlife."

And of course we would ride the Jungle Train. Not all the way to Limon for soul food and an overnight stay as we would have liked, because Harl had to be back at the hotel to refill his liquid oxygen after eight hours, but there was a shorter ride with a guide and a lunch that got him back in time. For the same reason we could not go to the southern tip and see rain forests, but we were happy enough with the Poas cloud forest.

The travel agent who booked the tours wasn't as nervous as the Visa people about things going wrong. When someone told her the wheelchair and oxygen were no problem, she believed them. When they told her we were booked, she believed them. I hounded her, making her double check. Even if the tours themselves could accommodate Harl, what about the shuttles from the hotel to the departure points? She said if there were problems with that, surely the tour people would have thought of it. I said, "*Check.*"

It was I who had become interested in Costa Rica, talking about perhaps even retiring there someday. Harl listened in the rapt way he listened to everything I said, obviously including himself in the retirement ideas. I winced, knowing that would be too late for him. And that I would not want to do it with him, go off to a strange country with no one to talk to.

Still, my whole impulse as I read about Costa Rica was to share it with him.

He had been wanting us to take another vacation for a long time. I had put it off over the summer, because of the expense. We were looking then at guided tours like the one we had taken to the Far East. Those would have given me company, people to talk to. But they were so elaborate, the places they went so expensive, that with my three children in college I really could not afford them. In Costa Rica we would not have a guide, but the place itself as I studied it seemed manageable. There was a lot of English spoken, and there was the Visa Assistance Center person there if we had an emergency.

Still, I had asked Harl if it might not be better to go someplace known and safe, perhaps back to Hawaii? He considered and shook his head no, smiling: "I'b *been* dere."

This was going to be a week of not talking at all, not with Harl because he could not talk and not with anyone else either because of the language barrier. But I felt up to it. There was something I liked about Harl's and my going off on this adventure alone.

I was still afraid to believe we would really go. Harl nudged me as we ate with Ray and Virginia, "Tell dem d'about Cotda *Wica!*" And he told his Wednesday morning aphasia group too. He pronounced the name always with the same enthusiastic emphasis: "Cotda *Wica!*"

But he too had a nervous edge as we planned, a persistent shadow that crossed his face and said he feared he would somehow not be able to go. He could have another crisis like the one that kept us from going to Russia, or the airlines could put us off a plane as they had done more than once on our other, shorter trips.

Sunday afternoons through the summer and on into September, I pushed him in his wheelchair around the park. His oxygen tank hung down between the handlebars behind him; on his lap he held the sack with our picnic in it. He stared at everything with the hunger of one who gets out in the world very little, the bicyclers, the volleyball players, the children.

Especially the children. There was a certain look he had for them, so rich and tender that no matter where we were, I had only to glance at him and see it flood his face, and would know without turning my own head to look that he had seen a child.

We found a table and unpacked our picnic, first sipping the wine that I had disguised in a rootbeer bottle. I joked about getting arrested, eyeing police cars across the park. I could even joke some about Harl with his wheelchair and oxygen: "I don't think they're going to want to take me when they get a load of you."

A rain storm came up, and I ran with the wheelchair halfway around the park to his building. He clutched the picnic sack in one hand and paper towels over his head with the other. When we reached shelter I flopped against the building, and we laughed together in exhilaration. Harl pointed upward to indicate his apartment and said, "Dyet's doe hab a *dwink*."

Yet I was feeling more burdened by him too than I had in a long time, although he was doing nothing unusual to burden me. I was restless, left him in the evenings sooner and spent more of my time with him reading.

We planned the trip on our Sunday mornings in bed. Harl turned the pages of the travel books, his hands pale on the blankets, pointing to pictures, marking restaurants. I wrote out an itinerary for us, checking it with him as I went. Arrive Thursday night. First day sleep late, after breakfast take a walking tour that is outlined in one of the books. Go to a Traditional Dinner With Folk Dancing at the hotel.

Second day a city bus tour in the morning and whatever is playing at the National Theater in the evening. Third day Jungle Train; I have spent hours making sure nothing will go wrong with that one. Fourth day free. We will sleep late again, walk to some place different for breakfast, and do whatever strikes our fancy.

Fifth day Poas Park, the cloud forest. Sixth day either a beach tour or another free day, depending on how we feel. That is the only one of the tours for which I have not signed us up in advance and talked at length with someone about the oxygen.

Seventh day home. Our plane leaves Thursday at seven a.m., so we will have to be at the airport at five. There and again in Miami and Atlanta, medical suppliers will come to provide oxygen. It will be a hard day.

We mapped it all out this final time on our last Sunday morning before leaving. Though we did not touch, I could feel a tension in Harl's body, that tightening of a muscle at the side of his neck that meant he was so hopeful about something he could hardly stand it.

Though we did not touch, I knew him that well.

I said what was in both our minds. "I hope we're really going. It's hard to let ourselves get excited when we're afraid something will happen and we won't get to go."

He nodded, apprehensive and smiling at the same time. He said, "It deems too wonderbul to be twue." The muscle in his neck jumped, and knotted into a hard lump.

* * *

We were all the way to Security, waiting to put my purse through the x-ray scanner, when I missed the little blue canvas bag with medications that Harl always carried carefully with him when he traveled. He had packed it; it was in my car the night before.

Stunned, we stared at each other. I had brought our bags in from the car that morning and set them in the front hall for a cab driver to help carry out. Harl had not seen the medication bag since I took it with his suitcase from his apartment the night before.

So this must have been my fault. But I could not remember the bag at all. Had I left it in the car? I knew Harl always carried it, so I didn't think I would have put it in the hall with the other bags. But perhaps I set it down there when I was going back to help Harl out, and the cab driver took it?

And then left it in the cab?

Harl could not go twenty-four hours without his heart medicines. But there was not time to go back. Should we go ahead and board, assuming we could get this taken care of somehow? Could Dr. Friedman call prescriptions to other states or countries?

It was seven a.m. I went to a phone and called David. If the bag was in my car or somewhere in my house, he could mail it to us. It must be possible to get emergency mail service to Costa Rica.

Miraculously, David answered. I was shaking with relief.

He would go and look for the bag. If he couldn't find it, he could mail us a second set of the medications that Harl kept at my house. He knew how to break in; he and Steve were both always losing their keys.

Holding the phone with my shoulder to my good ear, I dug out papers from the travel agency and read him the hotel's address. Fear was still turning my insides to noodles. Maybe we shouldn't go.

I told David I would call him again from Atlanta.

Harl sat still stunned in the snack bar where I had left him. Regaining confidence, I brought us coffee and omelets and told him David would mail us the medications.

Was he angry at me about this? It had to be my fault; Harl never forgot that bag. But I had been taking care of so many things, the bags and wheelchair and oxygen and going back to help him. It seemed natural to me that I might overlook one thing in the midst of all that, but I had always been more forgiving of my absentmindedness than Harl was. He did not say it was all right. He just kept on looking stunned.

The oxygen was waiting on the plane, that part at least going smoothly. I pulled out the extra plastic piece I had brought along to hook it to his trans-tracheal tube, smiling competently at the airline people who had not seen the trans-tracheal delivery before, showing them I had everything under control.

Harl sat in the window seat, beginning to look recovered. But for some reason the plane did not leave. After twenty minutes I started to read the book I carried to get me through this day. Then a man with an airline badge appeared and sat beside me.

He said, "I am going to have to ask you to leave this plane."

It had to be a mistake. I was too stupefied even to be scared. But I felt Harl go weak with fear beside me.

The man said that at Harl's litre flow he would have to start a second bottle of oxygen in flight. And there was an F.A.A. regulation against opening the bottles in flight.

I said we had flown lots of times, and he always started new bottles in flight. "And you knew his litre flow when we made these arrangements. This has been arranged for *months*."

He said he had been on the phone with F.A.A. for twenty minutes, and he was sorry but they would not bend. Maybe other airlines did sometimes do it, but it was a regulation and there would be a thousand dollar fine if anyone from F.A.A. saw them open a bottle in flight. "At two liters a minute we could get him to Atlanta on one bottle, but at three we can't. So I have to ask you to disboard."

Pulling from my purse the doctor letter that I had had the foresight to ask be written with a range instead of one number for the litre flow, I pushed it desperately at him. "Then we'll use two. This is his doctor's letter. It says two to four; we'll use two."

He was a nice enough man; he really did want us to be able to go. He seized the letter hopefully and carried it off with him. We waited scarcely breathing. Someone might still refuse us because the prescription they had said three. It was over just such small discrepancies that we had been put off before.

The man came back. He was smiling, so I knew it was all right. He handed the letter back to me and said, "It's okay. We'll use two."

Later I would figure out the problem had been with the

trans-tracheal delivery. Nasal canulas were attached to the oxygen bottles before they were put on board, so they did not have to be opened on board. Because Harl was not using the nasal canula, it would have taken a second or two to hook his tubing to the bottle. That was what F.A.A. prohibited.

He could have just used the nasal canulas. But no one had asked us.

But I had saved the trip for us, so now maybe Harl would not be angry with me about the medications. I pressed his hand as the plane took off, asking if he was happy.

A psychologist by training and temperament, he did not take questions about feelings lightly. He considered, then said resignedly, "No. I'm not appy."

I asked why. He gestured toward where the man had disappeared down the aisle. "Becud of dat appening."

And a moment later he said, still digesting it, "It was becud of *us* dat dey were d'yate."

I found I was not happy either. I said, "When we take off from Miami, that's when I'll believe we're going."

A page from my office was waiting in Atlanta. I called from a pay phone, Harl waiting on the plane. Davud had not found the bag but had found the second set of the medications. Only no one would mail them. Express services would not mail drugs and had no overnight service to Costa Rica anyway; delivery would take four days.

David had enlisted the help of the people at my office. They had called the V.A. Hospital hoping we could pick up replacement prescriptions in Miami. V.A. said their doctors could not prescribe for another state.

That noodles feeling again. I called Dr. Friedman, telling his nurse the problem. After a long wait Dr. Friedman came on. He was so calm that my knees wobbled with relief. "I'll just call the prescriptions either to Miami or Costa Rica. If you have long enough in Miami, get a cab and get to a drug store and have them call me."

We were supposed to have three hours, but we were already running late. And in Miami we still had to pay for the next flight's oxygen; that always took time. I could leave Harl in the care of the oxygen supplier, but he would be so frightened waiting for me that I could scarcely think of it. It would be better if I could find a drug store that would deliver to the airport. I called the Visa Assistance Center.

By now everyone there knew me. They were horrified. After all their work to make sure nothing went wrong for us, I was embarrassed to tell them this. They said they would get the prescription list from Dr. Friedman and try to get it filled in Costa Rica.

Crisis coping always made me high. I went back to where Harl waited pale with anxiety, and said with confidence born of adrenaline that I had talked to Dr. Friedman and it was going to be fine.

By Miami it was. Harl waited by a bank of seats while I called the Visa people again. They had reached their representative in Costa Rica, and he was going to meet us at the airport with the drugs.

Harl pointed to where his trans-tracheal tube connected at his throat, gesturing with the other hand as if pushing a button on an aerosol can. I understood at once. The aerosol spray he used to clean his tube up inside his throat was also inside that bag.

He said with a gesture of holding his hands about fourteen inches apart, "Tick."

Panic flooded me. Was he also missing the long wire stick he inserted up the tube to clean it? But no, he was telling me he *did* have the stick. "In my duit-tase. I hab duh *tick*."

I called the Assistance Center again to see if their Costa

Rica person could also bring us the cleanser.

The respiratory therapist in Miami was a young man in his middle twenties, very Cuban. He and I talked, Harl silent but listening in his wheelchair beside me. After awhile I brought us all drinks from a nearby lounge, looking surreptitiously at my watch and wondering how I would get through another hour.

Eventually I picked up a book and lost myself again, when the young man finally ran down.

He accompanied us all the way onto the plane, helping hook Harl's tubing to the airline's oxygen bottle. I offered him the plastic connecting piece I had brought with us, but that did not seem to be the problem. Something was wrong with the bottle; it would not work on the high litre flow. A flight attendant said it was better to use the lower litre flow anyway, "So we won't run out."

Harl had just paid three hundred dollars for six oxygen bottles, three each way, so he could have the high litre flow. But if I said anything, we might be put off. I nodded that the two liters would be all right, and waved goodbye to our young Cuban. He said he would make sure he was the one to meet us on our return trip.

Through the flight I kept checking Harl's hands. If they turned blue I would demand the higher litre flow, and they could use the plane's emergency oxygen if we ran out. But his hands were good, pink and warm.

He ordered two drinks, happily holding up two fingers, just as he had done on each of the other legs of our flight. I did not drink at all, because I had so much still to get through. I buried myself again in my book.

The San Jose Airport was terrifying, people who did not speak English pushing Harl away and motioning to me to go down another hall. It led to Customs; I stood in line and wondered if Harl had connected with the oxygen supplier. And how I was ever going to find him.

Everyone else seemed to have little cards that I did not. Now I remembered that our tour company was supposed to have given us tourist cards on the plane from Miami. But they had not.

I could not communicate with anyone. I would never see Harl again.

The man behind the window kept holding his hand out for the cards. I gave him everything I had, my boarding passes, my hotel registrations, my return tickets. I held my hands out in the helpless way Harl did; I pointed in the direction someone had taken him and said inanely, "Help."

The man went away and came back with the cards. I was sent on to Baggage, where our suitcases of course were not. I stood looking forlornly around me.

Someone said from behind me, "Mrs. Ruth?"

Our bags were already on a van, and Harl too. He was hooked to an oxygen tank, someone from the supply company on one side of him, a tour company person on the other. It was the Visa Assistance person who had found me.

Other travelers were in the seat behind us, to be taken to their hotels. I climbed on, and we took off as if everyone had been waiting on me. Even here everyone seemed to be in a hurry.

It was very dark. I put my hand on Harl's. If I had been frightened, I could not even imagine how frightened he had been.

The Visa man had the medications, though not the aerosol cleanser. We would have to look for that in a drugstore.

We pulled up at our hotel, in a dismayingly industrial-looking part of town. The oxygen man and Visa man both came in with us, through a courtyard that was pretty but to a room that was small and dark. The Visa man was the only one who spoke English.

In the room was a plug-in oxygenator, not the liquid oxygen I had requested. There were also two portable steel tanks; from what I knew of oxygen tanks, they would last us only about two hours each.

I asked again for the liquid oxygen, the Visa man translating. They did not know what I meant. They had never heard of it.

I told them we would at least need more of the portable tanks, so we could leave the hotel and do things. They talked; the Visa man translated for me that they would find as many tanks as they could.

They hooked Harl to the oxygenator, but they did not have a connecting piece to lengthen the tubing. I reached for the one I had brought, and remembered that our young Cuban had not given it back to me.

They were sweet people, as we had read that Costa Ricans were. A kindliness about them communicated itself even as they talked in Spanish to each other. Finally the Visa man translated for me. The supplier was closed for the night; they could not bring us the piece we needed until tomorrow. But they would bring it first thing tomorrow.

So for tonight Harl was leashed for want of a two-inch piece of plastic to two and a half feet of tubing.

He did laugh once, sitting on the edge of the bed by the machine after the two men had left, absorbing his predicament. This one he knew was not my fault. I had appealed to him as I insisted in unaccepting frustration to the two men that I *had* brought the very piece we needed. "Don't you remember I gave it to the supplier in Miami when he was working on that tank on the plane, and he dropped it in his pocket?" Harl nodded emphatically, remembering.

My frustration must be the frustration he felt about the medicines as well, seeing his own careful deliberate planning for himself shot down by someone else's moment of carelessness. But I had taken care of that, he had the medicines. So why was I still getting the impression he was angry at me?

He had not said he was, but he had not said he was not. And he was perfunctory about my success in getting the medicines replaced, not thanking me or smiling relief. Something about him was not his usual self.

But we were both very tired. He crawled into bed by the machine; I flipped out the light, and we both fell immediately asleep.

We woke to what seemed like mid-morning sunshine, at five a.m. I made coffee in the one-cup pot I carried with us all over the world, and sat in bed to share it with Harl while a second cup brewed. He sat propped on pillows in his clean white T-shirt, the plastic tube running from his throat to his oxygenator that breathed like a great beast beside him.

Mornings had always been our best times, sipping our coffee, reconnecting with each other.

It was Harl the consummate civilized man who got me into this tradition of drinking coffee in bed before considering anything as onerous as getting up, but it was I who expanded that to espresso coffees and bought the travel pot that let us keep that tradition everywhere in the world. He had given me repeated inordinate praise for that, gesturing at the coffee and the pot and me, his smile saying this was an incredibly wonderful thing I did.   Greedy for more of that, I sipped and handed the cup happily to him. *See this nice thing I do for you.*

I also showed him again the guidebook that mapped out our walking tour. Leisurely, "But no rush. Today we have all day."

But something was still wrong. Even at this early best time of the morning, he was not his usual warm appreciating self. He did not make a fuss over the coffee or gesture around in delight at the room, which though small and dark and not luxurious did have a character I thought he would appreciate. It was not like Harl to look on the bad side of things.

Maybe he would feel better when the oxygen supplier came back with more of the portable tanks and the plastic piece to lengthen his tubing. Maybe he was just still anxious about the oxygen.

We went downstairs to the courtyard cafe for breakfast, Harl pushing one of the two portable tanks on its cart in front of him. Whatever was bothering him did not keep him from his unwavering perfect grooming. He had showered and combed his hair; his shirt was starched and crisply pressed.

Breakfast perked him up some. No one loved good food more than Harl, and the courtyard cafe was lovely with ferns and white iron tables. But beyond it was the dismayingly busy city, not the oversized Santa Fe we had imagined but more like a Spanish New York. Cars honked and screeched; pedestrians swarmed the sidewalks.

But Harl had never before moped because a place was not up to his expectations. We still had our walking tour in front of us, and the Jungle Train, and the National Theater, and lots of native food. All the adventures we had been planning these last months pressed at me and made me excited in spite of Harl's lack of response. I exclaimed over the coffee that arrived strong and steaming with little pitchers of hot milk, prodding at Harl to share my delight. *Say it's all right, make me happy.*

These heavy steel oxygen tanks were going to be difficult with the wheelchair. They could not hang down behind it as

Harl's light liquid tank did, and they would last only two or three hours each as compared to twelve for the liquid. But there was no way to take an extra; we just could not get more than an hour away from our hotel.

I tried laying a tank across the bars of the chair, but it slid around and was hard for Harl to hold onto. We ended up standing it up between his legs; he gripped it with both hands and nodded that he was ready to go.

The sidewalks were rough for the chair, and so astonishingly crowded. Where could all these people be going? On each corner I stopped and pulled the guidebook from where it lay tucked next to Harl and studied it again to make sure we were going the right way. We were heading for the Mercado Central; the book said we would be "entering through the flower section." It did not say we would make our way there through screaming traffic.

Occasionally someone who spoke English saw me floundering on a corner with my guidebook and asked if he could help. One thing all the guidebooks said was that Costa Ricans are very nice people, helpful, and friendly to Americans. I thanked them and got my bearings again and pushed on, Harl saying nothing, gripping his oxygen tank firmly between his legs.

I worried that a bad bump could cause the tank to hit him in the mouth. At curbs I tipped him back and pressed the chair against my legs, sliding it down as gently as I could. Someone usually helped me get it up the other side.

One of the men who stopped to help said that with the wheelchair we were allowed to walk in the street. That was better, because the streets were not as crowded or bumpy. But some of them were so heavy with traffic that I did not dare walk there.

It was not what we had expected, but I was ready to like

it: the bustle, the nice people, the adventure. What kept me uncertain was Harl, his lack of expressions or gestures to show pleasure. I checked his oxygen tank and found with dismay that it had already dropped to almost empty. We would have to cut this walk short, turn around and go back.

Back in our room I called the supplier, asking when they were coming with more portable tanks. They arrived in a few minutes, two of them who did not speak English but smiled warmly as they produced the plastic connecting piece that would let Harl off his two-and-a-half-foot leash.

I sat on the edge of the bed with my Spanish dictionary, trying to explain our need for enough tanks for eight hours on the Jungle Train. And then for dinner after. I found the word for *hour*, pointing to the empty tank from our walk and holding up two fingers: "Dos horas."

So we would need at least six tanks for the day of the Jungle Train. They were flabbergasted, eyes widening as they grasped what I was saying. They were not sure they could come up with that many tanks.

After speaking for awhile in Spanish to each other, they turned back to me with smiles that said they thought they had a solution. One of them pointed to a tank and made a large gesture with his hands, indicating a huge tank.

Could such a tank be portable? I pointed to the small cart, then spread my own hands in the same large gesture, making my face a question.

He nodded eagerly, smiling, confident. In my dictionary he found "five" and "tonight," pointing to the words and himself and our room, spreading his hands again to show the huge oxygen tank. He would bring the tank to our room at five tonight.

We all kept laughing from the absurdity of trying to talk to each other. Except Harl, with whom I turned to share the lingering warmth when they left. He was not tuned in to it as I expected him to be; he sat back on the pillows with the same despondency he had been exhibiting all morning.

Usually he would have been interacting in his own way with these people, his smile making their eyes linger. Now he seemed not to think of doing that; he just sat back and watched as I handled everything, and people were not noticing as they usually did what a sweet alive person he was. Everyone was automatically looking only at me.

My own warmth fading as he failed to share it, I asked him what was wrong. "Why are you looking so depressed?"

He made a gesture rather like the shrug he used to do, suggesting *I don't know*, and also perhaps *Why not?*

A sudden anger ripped me. I said, "I don't want to spend a week with you looking like that. I mean it, I'd rather go home."

He gestured helplessly again, and suddenly there was a look on his face I had never seen there before: inward turning but also stubborn, belligerent almost.

What right did I have to demand happiness from him? If he was depressed, he was.

But I thought he might think it over and realize how he was affecting me. I went out and around a corner to a drugstore to look for the cleanser he still needed for his throat tube. We had passed the drugstore on our walk, but it was too crowded to get into with the wheelchair.

They had all kinds of other American products but not that one.

Remorse for what I had said was hitting me by the time I got back. That strange look that had crossed his face lingered with me. I put too much pressure on him to act happy; I had to let him show his depression if that was what he was feeling. I would pull back, let him be. I would not press him again.

But what was wrong? The way he had seemed to gesture, "Why not?" tended to confirm my feeling that he was disappointed with the place. That was not like him, but perhaps he had been thinking this would be his last vacation. Certainly this dark room and high traffic city were not much like the pictures he had stared at of Florence, Naples, Amsterdam.

So was he blaming me, because I had first started talking about Costa Rica? Or maybe he was blaming me for leaving his medications; maybe he was still preoccupied with that. His lack of effort to interact with me, to reassure me and make me feel better, was coming across as anger. Or at least I with my habitual slight paranoia would interpret it that way.

In one of the guidebooks I had circled the name of a clinic for emergency medical care, showing Harl as he watched beside me in the security of my bed back home. All this had seemed so much safer then. Harl had been so happy then.

Cotda Wica!

A medical clinic would surely have the cleanser or some similar product. My eyes turned to Harl as I dialed the number. He would see how I cared for him, the attention that I gave to this.

The woman who answered spoke no English. She conveyed that no one there spoke any English. *Lo siento*.

Harl and I looked at each other, I baffled and, because I thought he was blaming me, nervous; he--flat, perfunctory. I thought angry, but possibly more scared.

We were going before lunch to the tour company's office to confirm our reservations for Poas Park and the Jungle Train. I said we could ask them to suggest another drugstore.

After lunch Harl lay down and I put on my red raincoat

and went out. Even when I was with him I fantasized a lot, distancing myself from the not-talking through the imaginings of my mind. Away from him, energized by rebellion and relief, I fantasized even more.

And I absorbed more of this busy bustling city, beginning to like it. Streets were narrow and buildings dingy, but there was nothing seedy about the people. Though I knew from my reading they were a relatively poor people, they were astonishingly well-dressed. Young women tripped about under umbrellas in stylish short skirts and high heels; men wore crisp smartly cut shirts; everyone had clean hair. They reminded me of Harl with his continuing perfect grooming; there was a pride about them I thought he would appreciate.

The rain had been late today. Harl had fallen asleep before it started, commenting dourly, "It did't eben wain." When I came back he lay on his back still snoring lightly. I struggled to open the room's one small window that was by his bed, so he could get the breeze and the good rain smell. The window was wedged somehow; it would not open.

He opened his eyes and looked at me foggily. I gave up on the window and settled for telling him happily, "It's raining like *hell*."

His eyes turned to the window, but without a lot of response. I just could not cheer him up.

Halfway through the Saturday morning city tour, he started a dry coughing. My eyes swung to him, across the bus aisle from me with the five-foot high oxygen tank wedged between us. "Why are you coughing?"

He shrugged.

We had still not found the cleanser; he had not cleaned his tube in two days. It was odd how I was able to keep forgetting about this. Now I explained it to the tour guide, asking since he spoke English if we could hire him to come to a clinic with us. Why hadn't I thought to talk to the guide about this right at the beginning of the tour, instead of only after Harl started coughing? Perhaps my escape into habitual daydreaming had consequences of which I was unaware; perhaps I was really not functioning very well.

The guide was young and congenial, smartly dressed like all these people. He said he would take us to the clinic.

First he called them from a pay phone at the hotel, speaking to me in English and translating into the phone in Spanish. Harl waited behind us, looking wretched. His huge oxygen tank beside him was fastened with chains to its wheeled cart, which surprisingly was not hard to push.

The guide put a hand over the mouthpiece and said, "Why don't you go to the desk first and ask to talk to the hotel doctor. Every hotel has a doctor."

The doctor had a call back to me in five minutes. He spoke English; I described the trans-tracheal surgery and told him the product we needed. He said, "We don't have that procedure here. But I will be over in thirty minutes, and either I will have your product or I will be able to tell you what to do."

We waited in our room, relief already making me giddy. But why hadn't I thought of the hotel doctor myself, yesterday? Perhaps I did not clearly know that every hotel had a doctor, but I certainly knew it was a possibility. The blame must indeed lie partly with this foggy daydreaming state I got into, my escape from the not-talking.

But I did not think I could stop that. It was what enabled me to bring Harl on a trip like this. It was what had gotten me through these last six years.

Dr. Rodriguez was dashing in a pink polo shirt inscribed in English, "Playboy." He seemed very competent; he looked at the throat tube and said it could be cleaned without the special cleanser. "It wouldn't be sterile in there anyway. He can just use the stick, or use Phisohex if he wants." We had Phisohex.

He left, urging us to call him again if we had any other problems. Harl went into the bathroom to clean his tube.

Rain was starting up for the second time, our second full day here. How could I be this relieved, when I had not been aware of being that anxious? Harl came out and lay down; I put on my red raincoat and went to walk in the rain again, looking not for drugstores this time, but for places I could wheel him to for lunch.

Everything was American. Harl held his oxygen tank with one hand and our umbrella low over his head with the other, so I could see over it as I wheeled him to a *Soda* for their lunch special: two pieces of fried chicken, French fries, a tortilla and a Coke, for $1.29. The tortilla was what made it Central American.

We laughed, looking bewilderedly out at the stream of pedestrians on the sidewalk. I said, "I've figured it out. This *is* the native food."

It was the best time we had, rain smells blowing in through the open front door, Harl damp in his red wheelchair laughing over his plate of fast food. Our connection still working, still there.

* * *

The Jungle Train was good too, Harl and I facing each other in the small balloon-decorated car, the huge oxygen tank wedged behind his seat. The guide was a warmly smiling black woman from Limon who paid Harl special attention.

She said the oxygen was no problem, just no problem at all. People brought him things, snacks, drinks, a good box lunch. He smiled at them in more of his usual way and said, "Dant dou." He did not have the abject despondent look that he had worn for so much of this trip.

Yet there was a deep sadness in him. I was not sure how I knew; I just knew. It was in something fragile in the set of his mouth, or the extra gentle way he said, "Dant dou."

I snapped pictures out the window, watched the guide or the countryside, looked back at him and every time saw that sadness and did not know what to say. So I said nothing.

Harl said gently as we got off, motioning to the guide, "Tip her *weal* well."

As we shared our cup of coffee in bed the next morning, he said with a similar undercurrent of deep feeling, "Our batation is 'af ober."

It was the first time he had expressed anything positive about this vacation. I was so convinced he was disappointed, and felt so bad about that, that I could not deal with it directly. This might have been a time to ask him, more gently than last time, what was bothering him. Instead I smiled over at him and said more guardedly, "I know. It's going too fast."

He nodded, then said hopefully and unexpectedly, "In duh pwing maybe we tan doe to D'yondon and *Paris*."

He was so sick, I knew he would not take another trip. But I played along, helping him deny. Embellishing even, to make it seem more real. "I think maybe not Paris, because" -- gesturing toward the many-sized oxygen tanks lining one wall--"we need a lot of help, and you always hear that the French are not very nice. I think I might be afraid to go where people aren't helpful. But I think we could handle London."

He said eagerly, with a movement of his arm, "D'yondon and I'deland!"

Almost as if it were really going to happen, I as eagerly agreed. "Yes! There are some good deals to London and Ireland. We can go with a tour that time."

Maybe it would even happen. If the lung disease slowed down, if he was not institutionalized by then. For just a moment I could see us, disembarking in another airport, Harl happy in his red wheelchair. The two of us ready to do London and Ireland.

The vision faded. I wondered if it did for him too, if his own deep true heart would tell him it could never happen.

* * *

The guide for the Poas Park tour came looking for us in the lobby, and did a double take when he saw the large oxygen tank. "We're not taking *that*, are we?"

Harl sat despondent by the tank, his canvas rain hat on his head, raincoat and umbrella on his lap. Our guidebook said to bring rain gear to Poas.

Just yesterday I had spent an hour on the phone with the tour company, talking about the oxygen tank. I said, "They must have told you. I've talked to them about this lots of times. They said it wasn't any problem."

He said, not unkindly really, but tactlessly, "We'll try it. But it *is* a problem."

We were seated across an aisle from each other, in small seats just behind the driver where neither of us could hear the guide well. Was it the comment about the oxygen tank that had Harl *so* depressed? He stared vacantly out the window, so unhappy that his lips trembled and his eyes had no life at all. This had to be more than a reaction to the tactless comment, a continuation of whatever had been bothering him this whole trip.

Helpless, I stared out my own window and lost myself again in daydreaming.

This was not the nature tour we had expected, just a look at Poas Volcano and a farmhouse lunch and back to the hotel. They walked us up a short hill to look down into the volcano, the guide on one side of Harl and I on the other. I had the oxygen turned up to five, but he still had to stop every few steps. At the top he stared down into the steaming crater, saying nothing. I had never liked geysers; they gave me a bad feeling.

I kept checking Harl's hands. His face was strained but not gray, and his hands were still pink. His color had been really good this whole trip; I had told him a couple of times that I thought the extra exercise must be good for him. Each time he threw me a strange look, and said nothing.

Back on the bus the guide said, "Let's have a hand for Mr. Young. Because he is really brave to do this."

I smiled over at Harl and clapped with the rest, but he just glanced up in surprise and got tears in his eyes and looked back out his window. He had not even smiled; he was in the lowest mood I had ever seen him in.

After we got back, I sat by Harl on the bed and looked again at what our guidebook said about Poas. A cloud forest, thirty-eight species of bird life. I showed it to Harl, who had not answered me when I said something about the Poas tour being disappointing. Showing him it wasn't my fault, that he should not be angry at me.

Lying back down, withdrawing again into my daydream. Feeling that he was blaming me.

Helping him into the shower as I did each day, a hand on his pale bony elbow. The scars from his heart surgeries ran in deep craters down and across his chest; his abdomen was white and mottled. He still had the slight pear shape of a leprechaun, but he was so thin that his legs were little more than sticks, bottom shriveled to nearly nothing. How could I love his body this consciously, yet be feeling so reluctant to initiate sex with him? We had not made love this whole trip; it was the one thing I did not offer him.

But why not? Perhaps I was angrier or more hurt by how he was acting than I had been letting myself realize. Because I felt he had a right to his mood and was trying not to pressure him, I was stifling my own disappointment.

And he had not initiated lovemaking either, although we both had surely expected we would do it on this trip. I listened to the sound of his shower, hoping it was only my imagination that whether or not I initiated sex at this time was important to him. He saw so much evidence of my care, the time I spent on the phone making arrangements for him, the oxygen, green tanks of I-love-you lining a wall of the room. Not making love in Costa Rica didn't mean we wouldn't again, we would when he was home and rested and in a better mood.

* * *

Our last day. We passed on the beach tour and chose a free day after all. Or Harl did; I always did what he wanted. But I was happy with it.

I pushed him several blocks to a restaurant our guidebook suggested for breakfast, wheeling his chair neatly up to the table, looking up the menu items in my Spanish dictionary and reading them to him. Ham and eggs, bacon and eggs, French toast. One of our tour guides had given me the name of a dinner restaurant for real Central American food; we were going there tonight.

I pushed the wheelchair back toward the hotel, stopping at a bookstore where I bought a *Tico Times*. Harl looked at it and wanted a copy of his own for a souvenir. On down the street we went into an art gallery, and he bought a painting for his apartment. I wondered where he would find a free square inch of wall space to put it.

The rain began. I made him a drink, put on my red raincoat and went out. He was still acting depressed, looking morosely out the window. I couldn't wait to get away from him.

This time I went east, and after several blocks came to the Parque Espana. We had not located this before; someone had told us there wasn't a good park in walking distance.

I found a bench and sat down looking into the park, water running off my umbrella. Even in this much rain the sidewalks were full of people.

I was quite proud of myself for my handling of this trip. How changed I was from the time of our Far East trip five years before, when I had spent the whole time wondering how I could get through it. And we had other people with us then.

Harl wasn't even on *oxygen* then.

All our earlier trips, even those from before Harl's stroke, I had experienced as being done to me. Only this one I had done myself, guidebook and dictionary in hand. And I had done it with the incredible challenge of Harl's condition, the wheelchair and oxygen, the not-talking.

A week in a strange country with the not-talking, and I had faced it calmly. I had even had rather a good time.

I said to myself, *What a woman.*

Yet I would not have done it without Harl. Picture the scene with him out of it, the hotel room behind me empty, no wheelchair to push, no Harl across a table as I read from my dictionary, and I did not want to be in it either. For all the difficulty in traveling with him, it was the communication I had with him that made my own pleasure possible.

So why was I again having this persistent half thought that I might like him to die?

That thought was what I puzzled over as I watched the rain run off my umbrella. It was not what I really wanted; otherwise the thought itself would not frighten me as it did. The fright came from my irrational but probably only human feeling that my thinking this made it more likely to happen.

My heart twisted with the fright. I didn't mean it; I didn't want him to die.

Where then did that thought I so feared and hated come from?

There was the horror of what I saw in store for him, the slow horrible drowning in his own lungs. And I knew I saw his dying as the only thing that would release me from his care. So perhaps this was as simple as an only natural wish for some release, for both of us.

Because I had lived with it so long, perhaps too I was overlooking how really terrible not talking is. Or repressed the terribleness, so that it surfaced as a death wish.

That was part of it, but I felt there was more. Perhaps what I still denied to myself, the loss of him in spite of the sweetness we still had: the joy we had taken in our conversation, the astonishing connection between us, talking for whole mornings in bed together with never a failing of our interest in each other.

Did I need to acknowledge a part of me that wanted that again?

Most of the time I felt so bound to Harl by what we had been through, the terribleness as well as the sweetness, that I thought I could not have another intense relationship after him. But probably that wasn't realistic. Those who love, love again.

But certainly not soon. I looked carefully and could not find in myself even a fantasy that such a connection could happen again soon, if Harl died. For the near future all I could see was a long stretch of loneliness, an absence of Harl that I could not even imagine.

So that possible far-off future love could not explain this baffling present wish for him to die.

I was ruthless with myself and would consider anything, even something crass. I was named as Harl's beneficiary on some insurance policies, and for some additional money under his will. But I would put that away for the future; it would make no change in my life right now. It would be security, but there was as much security in knowing I would have it as in having it. The money was not it.

An anger then. Was there something for which I was so angry at Harl that I wanted to kill him?

Perhaps for the not-talking, for which perhaps I still unconsciously blamed him. It is impossible for the unconscious mind to believe that an adult person who always talked before cannot talk now; it cannot help but hate him for that silence.

But there seemed to be something else, something more connected to his illness.

I stared through the rain into the park, trying to read there the riddles of my own heart. I had been through an illness before, with my mother. Was this in some way a replay of that?

For dying, was I angry enough at her to kill her?

The rain was letting up, and I was beginning to be distracted by happier thoughts. It was still early. I could hurry back to the hotel and bring Harl here in his wheelchair, let him sit awhile in this park that I wished I had found for him sooner.

My steps picked up until I was almost running, bursting into the room with rain running off my coat and hair to tell him about the park. "If the rain stops by five, I could take you there before we go to dinner. Do you want to go?"

He was still drinking, here in this small dark room thinking his own thoughts even as I sat on the park bench thinking mine. He made a slight helpless gesture, not really excited. I made myself a drink, and the rain kept on, and we did not talk again about going to the park.

* * *

Miami, and our oxygen supplier was not there. A man from the airlines stayed with us, letting Harl stay hooked to the airplane's bottle. Technically that bottle was not supposed to leave the plane, but they could hardly pull him off it.

The bottle was almost empty. I turned the litre flow down to two. Harl huddled with hunched shoulders, watching as I telephoned the Visa people.

They got on the phone with the supplier, who said their person was at the airport. There had been some problem in Customs. Now perhaps he did not know where to find us. We tried a page; no answer.

After nearly an hour of paging and phone calling, and with the bottle from the plane showing empty, I spotted the same young Cuban who had met us here before, pushing a tank of liquid oxygen and holding another under his arm. I dropped the phone and went after him, calling from yards away.

He was so upset that at first all he could do was rant at the man from the airline, while I took a tank from him and hooked Harl to it myself. Harl took a deep relieved breath and nodded to me that it was working.

Our young Cuban had been detained in Customs by the very airline on which we flew, apparently out of the anti-Cuban sentiment in Miami. They had claimed to think he got off the plane from Costa Rica, and to think the oxygen tanks might contain drugs.

He had told them Harl's name and flight number and that he needed continuous oxygen. They would not radio the plane to verify.

I said to Harl as we took off from Miami, "I'm so tired. I wish we didn't still have a layover in Atlanta." I did not know how I could endure that layover, three more hours of not talking. We had been at the San Jose airport at five, and I had been awake since three.

Harl rolled his eyes toward me and said nothing. He had been dozing on the plane, unusual for him. I continued to feel he was angry at me, blaming me for his disappointment with this whole trip.

I think during sleep deprivations the old reptilian brain is more in control. I hated Harl; I remembered every bad thing he had ever done. I couldn't wait to be rid of him, away from this mood of his that had spoiled my vacation.

I wouldn't mind the Atlanta layover so much if I didn't have to be with him. I just wanted to be away from him.

* * *

David waited at the gate in Denver, handsome, cheerful. He pushed the wheelchair, helped with the bags, helped Harl who had to use the restroom. With help I felt suddenly collapsed. I did not know how I had ever gotten through this.

I would have to leave the wheelchair in Baggage and come back the next day. David's car was not big enough for everything we had.

Should I take Harl to my house for the night? So we could wake up together in the morning and talk about our trip? We had not talked about what we were going to do tonight.

I told David to drive us to Harl's apartment. I wanted to be away from him. Away from him, away from him, away from him.

As I tried to help him out with his oxygen tank, he was motioning to me to wait. But I didn't see why, so I kept on.

He screamed in pain. The tank had somehow hurt his hand.

I still could not see how. I stood back watching him shake his hand, his face contorted. To David, but within earshot of Harl, I said hopelessly, "I'm always hurting him!" and walked around and stood alone behind the car.

Once at a restaurant in Costa Rica I had knocked an oxygen tank over on Harl's foot. He had cried out and grimaced that same way then.

David got Harl out. I walked past him and ahead with David to the elevator, waiting there as Harl pushed his oxygen cart along behind us.

He sank down on his sofa. I hooked him to his stationary oxygen tank, and turned and looked at him.

David was taking his bags to the bedroom, asking what else he could do to help. With a despair that had little to do with the practical problems of traveling with him, my week of dealing with the medications and the wheelchair and the oxygen, and everything to do with the mood he had been in for that week, I went out without saying goodbye.

* * *

Saturday morning I called him. He answered at once, sounding good. I asked, "Are you rested?"

He said, "Eah! Are dou?"

I said, "I'm rested some. But I'm still tired. I don't want to go out tonight."

He made a sound of what seemed to be agreement.

A few minutes later he called back, still sounding cheerful. He wanted me to bring the spare set of his medications from my house. In that odd formal way he had, "If you sould 'appen to dwop *by*."

I paused, not ready to see him yet. But he had to have the medications; he must be almost out of those he got in Costa Rica. And the way I had left him might have made him fear I would stop taking care of him. I would not, not even as I was feeling just now, not ever. I wanted him to know that, so I said, "I have your wheelchair too, and the picture you bought and some other things of yours that were in my suitcase. So I'll come by with all of it sometime this afternoon."

He said, "O'tay."

I got there at five, pushing the wheelchair with the medications and the other things I had brought. He was wearing overalls, drinking a beer and watching a game. He looked at me sharply, as if checking out something.

I exclaimed at how different he looked in his overalls than in the more formal clothes I had been seeing him in all week. But he had the game on. I asked, "Do you want to watch the game?" He nodded. So I did not sit down.

But I turned at the door, smiling back at him with my usual difficulty separating. He leaned forward and smiled and waved in the comical way he always did, and I waved back as I always did.

In the hall my discouragement at once returned. I did not want to be with him yet. I might not want to be with him this whole weekend.

But what else would I do? My life was so centered around Harl that it was hard to fill even one weekend without him.

I puttered, cleaning, on Sunday going for a walk. Thinking I would not break down and go to Harl just because I had nothing better to do.

I should call him, though. But then, he could call me too. By evening I was oddly depressed, still thinking I would call him soon but putting it off as I started to pay bills.

The phone rang. I practically dived for it. How could I so deceive myself, thinking I did not want to be with him, when I realized in this split second that I had been waiting all day for him to call *me*? And now that he had I could still go over and see him. It was only seven; we could still have drinks and dinner. I would ask him about his seeming disappointment with the trip, and he would be surprised. He would make gestures to indicate his stroke and the oxygen and all the problems, saying maybe he was a little bummed out about all that. But our vacation--he would put a hand on mine and smile his rich smile at me; he would say our vacation was *wonderbul*.

A man said, "This is the Park Lane."

And as I came to my feet with a great lurch of my heart thinking he was going to say Harl was having an emergency and they were calling him an ambulance, he said, "Mr. Young has passed away," and he said something else too after that, but I did not hear it because of my own screaming.

II

My children flank me in my pew, startling in their grown-up clothes. Their love has wrapped me like bright velvet all this week since Harl died, David driving over that night to stay with me, Cathryn flying home. Steve is taping the service. He wears a tie borrowed from David and his best white shirt, from which his wrists stick out.

We are in a Denver University chapel, small and beautiful. The flowers are mostly bright; I like that and think I will never send anything white to a funeral. Cindy and Fredd and I have asked the organist to play a medley of gospel songs. It is the best music we can think of to say who Harl was.

Paul Robeson singing out in rich baritone, *Swing Low, Sweet Chariot*. Harl with a hand to his mouth as he breaks into tears.

It was not even a five-minute drive from my house to his apartment. Gripping the steering wheel, crying *no*. Running (yet I know there is no use in running now; some part of me still hopes crazily for another near miss, but I know this is not one), his door ajar, a woman whom I will learn is the medical examiner seated at his table but I do not ask who she is, I run to the bedroom and it is empty and then to the bathroom, and there he is.

A plunge off the toilet, hands still at his sides, no struggle. But he has bled where his head hit the floor, face down in a pool of blood. The woman runs to my side, but I am good and will not make a scene. I hear her asking if I am his daughter. I cannot answer, I kneel and put a hand on his leg. It does not feel as cold as I expect. I want to nuzzle into his neck as I did not do the last chance I had, but I know it will be cold, so I do not.

He looks so helpless, and there is nothing I can do to help him.

The woman and I sit at his table. She says they often find cardiac patients this way. "Just as they are about to expire they feel that they need to move their bowels, and then they go." We realize it must have happened the night before, probably just a couple of hours after I saw him, because his Sunday paper still lies outside his door, and the Lifeline was activated when it was not reset for twenty-four hours. He has been lying here dead all day, while I listened for my phone to ring.

People come to take him out. From where I sit I see one of them lifting him by his ankles. I start to go and look again, because I am plagued by unreality and need to see things, but the woman runs out and stops me. She does not want me to see his face. She says I will see him again when they get him cleaned up.

They leave me alone, a door closing with a soft thud. I go to his bed, and press my face into the pillow that still smells so strongly of him, and cry and cry.

Steve and Cathryn whisper. They change places so Cathryn can hold my hand, from where my diamond ring shoots light. The organist slides into *The Old Rugged Cross*.

This is a service only, no casket. At some later time we

will inter the ashes. Before his stroke, before I knew him even, Harl joined a memorial society and requested cremation, but I know nothing of what he might have wanted beyond that. Through all this time of his failing, we have not talked about it. I thought he was too emotional, not able since the stroke to distance himself. But now I wonder if I could have helped him more with what he had to face. All those summer hours that he sat in contemplation on his balcony, wouldn't he have contemplated his own death?

So I don't mind dying so mutz.

But he did mind; he fought it until he couldn't anymore.

The people who have come today want to honor Harl, their memories of him. Once I imagined standing up at such a service and asking anyone who had not seen him in six years to leave, but now I have forgotten all that and am grateful for everyone who comes. I keep turning my head to see who is here, who bears this witness with me.

The minister has met with us to talk about Harl, about what we want him to say. Donna and Jeane are so happy with him that it makes them cry, because he is so nice and so thoughtful.

He talks of Harl's love of life. "I am sure Harl Young is a person I would have very much cherished as a friend....He was a scholar and a teacher, a counselor and a caregiver, a man of courage and determination....Six years ago Harl suffered a stroke that totally changed his life. But he didn't give up on life, he didn't quit. He said, `There is still a life to live.'"

He goes on to say something about me, about my making it possible for Harl to live the last years of his life with courage and determination. I watch him fascinated, as if he has something I need, an answer to something. What he says is what everyone has been saying to me, how happy it must make me to know I did so much to make Harl's life good for him. This is what anyone would naturally say, what I until now would have said to someone in similar circumstances, but I notice it is not what I want. What I want them to say is what Harl gave me back, the warmth of him, the quick tears, the sweet eager smile. Letting me believe I made him happy.

I have never been happier.

Donna and Jeane and Cindy and Fredd have been with me all this week; with their constant company I have been able to stave off some of the worst of what I will feel.

I have not yet pulled the box of his ashes from where it lies wrapped in his bathrobe on a closet shelf, and hugged it to my chest, and cried his name.

But I have felt the deep fear that hits in my stomach each morning as I wake, and makes me once again unable to eat. First I think I must be afraid of how I am going to feel. Then I perceive something else, the fear of having to manage in the world without Harl to take care of me.

I am not ready for that twist, that turn of the screw. Even I thought it was I who took care of Harl. I did not realize until now how much he still took care of me, in the emotional way that was the only way left to him. How am I going to live without his rapt attention to me, his crying for happiness when I come in with pieces of silverware, his distressed patting of my hand when I tell him about business problems?

I wish I had seen this sooner, this care he took of me, so I could have told him what it meant to me. He was so humble after the stroke; he would have wept at hearing that. But I tell myself he knew. It was so much what Harl was, the feeling giving caretaking man. It was what he lived for those six years.

The minister asks if some of us here would like to speak, to share something of our memories of Harl. I was nervous in the planning of this part because I was afraid no one would say anything. But after a short awkward silence, an old friend from Harl's days at the V.A. Hospital stands up.

Irv of the endless wit, whom Harl loved. He tells about his first arrival in Denver, and Harl meeting him at the airport in his red Triumph. Harl took him at once in the top-down Triumph to the foothills (now a shopping center) to show him the mountains.

Irv says, "That was Harl's idea of welcoming me to Denver. And for a boy from New York--well, I could have gone home *then*."

A man from the aphasia group stands up. I have invited the whole group, these people who were Harl's friends in the last months he lived. The school has opened up special parking for them, but many still felt they could not physically manage coming. I know how upset they are, how upset Harl would have been if one of them had died. I realize most people with these limitations would not take off as Harl and I did to Costa Rica, and ride the Jungle Train.

The man says, movingly because he does not talk very well, "Harl always wanted to go to a *party*."

Cotda Wica!

The wife of another of the group members stands up. There are tears in her eyes; her husband weeps beside her. She says, "My husband and I will always remember his warm eyes."

It is she and the others from the aphasia group who really matter to me. Everyone else has come in memory of a Harl of before the stroke; to them it is as if he died six years ago.

I am not angry at them anymore. But there is a fierceness in me; I want them to know about the Harl they missed, the grace and joy and sweet strength of him, and the beauty in those November days.

I d'yuv you.

Postscript

For months I had terrible dreams; I am being taken to a concentration camp, everything is black and grey and barbed wire and someone says over a loudspeaker that I am wearing lipstick and have been seen running my fingers through my hair; that is not allowed here. Harl is with me in his red wheelchair, that and my lipstick the only color in the dream. I tell him we have to escape, this place is crazy and terrible and we cannot stay. He stares back at me, mute, waiting as he always did. Harl.

Or I have left someone in a concentration camp, an elderly woman who stares at me from a wheelchair and does not reproach me. I cannot remember why I left her; I remember that I love her and that she trusts me and is completely dependent on me. I am dismayed, horrified; she is frail and I know she has surely died in the short time I have left her there, but I am going back to try to find her. I am so frightened she will be dead that I wake up, and know it is Harl who is dead.

And someone else too, the dream that is not a dream but what really happened. The five of us stand at an airport fence, watching our father help our mother onto the plane. It is raining; we are bedraggled in our cotton jackets, saying nothing. Our mother moves very slowly. I am twelve and know she is in bad pain and going to a Christian Science home somewhere, but I still think she will turn around at the top of the stairs and look back at us.

Debbie runs forward and presses her face against the fence. She is two and also expects her mother will look back.

They vanish inside the plane. She did not look back.

Not the death, then, but the time before. The time of withdrawal from what one must leave, five little girls or one helpless lover, the withdrawal they will never understand. And should not, because it violates the earth's earliest promise, the good rich mother promise: the attention, the warm smiles, the welcoming as one comes in. The turning to look back.

I was getting close to this as I sat puzzling on my park bench in Costa Rica, the root of the long plaguing anger that seems now mysteriously taken from me. But I stopped too soon then and did not see--in spite of, because of having been through this before, that nothing could make Harl behave the way he was behaving, except that he was dying.

Instead I latched onto a hope for bringing those good things back, run back to the hotel and push Harl here in his wheelchair, and then maybe he will be happy and make me happy again.

He would not make me happy again, but he has done this for me: waited to die until he saw me again, so that my last memory is not of leaving him in silent despair after Costa Rica, but of our smiling at each other, waving goodbye.

So that we have not left each other as my mother left me.

So that I will survive.
